Diabetics a
Cholesterol

Dr. Christie Barron

Disclaimer

Please keep in mind that the content in this book is solely for educational purposes. The information offered here is said to be reliable and trustworthy. The author makes no implication or intends to offer any warranty of accuracy for particular individual cases.
Before beginning any diet or lifestyle habits, it is recommended that you contact a knowledgeable practitioner, such as your doctor. This book's material should not be utilized in place of expert counsel or professional guidance.
The author, publisher, and distributor expressly disclaim all liability, loss, damage, or danger incurred by persons who rely on the information in this book, whether directly or indirectly.
All intellectual property rights are retained. This book's information should not be replicated in any way, mechanically, electronically, photocopying, or by any other methods accessible

Table of Contents

Why This Book Will Solve Your Problem

Are you tired of navigating the intricate landscape of managing diabetes and high cholesterol? Have you found it challenging to strike a balance between delicious, satisfying meals and maintaining a health-conscious lifestyle? If these questions resonate with you, then you're not alone. The journey to better health can be overwhelming, but fear not – our "Cookbook for Diabetics and High Cholesterol" is here to guide you through a transformative culinary experience that transcends the mundane notion of dietary restrictions.

Why this Cookbook?

1. **Tailored Nutrition for Optimal Health:** Our cookbook is crafted with a deep understanding of the nutritional needs of individuals managing diabetes and high cholesterol. Each recipe is a careful blend of ingredients that not only satisfy your taste buds but also contribute to your overall well-being.

2. **Balanced and Flavorful:** Gone are the days when "healthy" meant sacrificing flavor. Our recipes are a testament to the marriage of health-conscious choices and indulgent taste. From Quinoa Breakfast Bowls to Baked Garlic Herb Chicken Thighs, each dish is a celebration of wholesome ingredients coming together in perfect harmony.

3. **Scientifically Grounded:** Every recipe is meticulously designed to align with the principles of managing diabetes and high cholesterol. We've consulted with nutrition experts to ensure that each

ingredient serves a purpose in promoting heart health and glycemic control.

4. **Diverse Options for Every Meal:** Breakfast, lunch, and dinner – we've got you covered. With a variety of 75 recipes, you can break free from the monotony of repetitive meals and indulge in a diverse array of dishes that cater to your specific dietary needs.

How Will This Cookbook Solve Your Problems?

1. **Blood Sugar Management:** Our recipes are curated to help stabilize blood sugar levels, offering a well-rounded approach to diabetes management. Through a thoughtful selection of low-glycemic ingredients and balanced nutritional profiles, you can enjoy meals that won't cause unwarranted spikes.

2. **Cholesterol Control:** High cholesterol doesn't mean bidding farewell to delicious meals. Our cookbook emphasizes heart-healthy choices, incorporating ingredients proven to support cholesterol management. From omega-3 rich salmon to fiber-packed legumes, each recipe contributes to a heart-friendly diet.

3. **Culinary Empowerment:** Forget the notion of restrictive diets. Our cookbook empowers you to take charge of your health without compromising on the joy of eating. Discover the pleasure of preparing and savoring meals that align with your health goals.

4. **Education on Ingredients:** Gain a comprehensive understanding of the nutritional benefits of each ingredient. We provide insights into why certain foods are advantageous for

diabetes and cholesterol management, enabling you to make informed choices beyond the cookbook.

Embark on a culinary journey that transcends the limitations of health-conscious cooking. Our "Cookbook for Diabetics and High Cholesterol" is not just a collection of recipes; it's your ally in achieving a balanced, flavorful, and healthful lifestyle. Take the first step towards a healthier you – where every meal is a step closer to well-being. Your journey to culinary and health excellence begins here.

RECIPES

Quinoa Breakfast Bowl with Berries

Intro: This Quinoa Breakfast Bowl is a powerhouse of nutrition, combining protein-packed quinoa with fresh, antioxidant-rich berries. It's a delightful and energizing start to your day.

Total Prep Time: 20 minutes

Ingredients:
- 1 cup cooked quinoa
- 1/2 cup mixed berries (strawberries, blueberries, raspberries)
- 1 tablespoon honey
- 1/4 cup Greek yogurt
- 1 tablespoon chia seeds
- 1 tablespoon chopped almonds

Instructions:
1. In a bowl, layer cooked quinoa.
2. Top with mixed berries and drizzle honey over the berries.
3. Add a dollop of Greek yogurt.
4. Sprinkle chia seeds and chopped almonds over the top.
5. Mix well before enjoying.

Nutritional Information: (Per serving)
- Calories: 350
- Protein: 12g
- Carbohydrates: 45g
- Fiber: 7g
- Fat: 15g

Avocado and Tomato Omelette

Intro: This Avocado and Tomato Omelette is a savory delight, combining the creaminess of avocado with the freshness of tomatoes. It's a nutrient-packed breakfast that keeps you fueled throughout the day.

Total Prep Time: 15 minutes

Ingredients:
- 2 eggs
- 1/2 avocado, sliced
- 1/2 cup cherry tomatoes, halved
- Salt and pepper to taste
- 1 tablespoon olive oil
- Fresh herbs for garnish (optional)

Instructions:
1. Whisk eggs in a bowl and season with salt and pepper.
2. Heat olive oil in a pan over medium heat.
3. Pour whisked eggs into the pan.
4. Add avocado slices and halved cherry tomatoes on one side.
5. Once the edges are set, fold the omelette in half.
6. Cook until eggs are fully set.
7. Garnish with fresh herbs if desired.

Nutritional Information: (Per serving)
- Calories: 280
- Protein: 14g
- Carbohydrates: 10g
- Fiber: 5g
- Fat: 20g

Greek Yogurt Parfait with Nuts and Seeds

Intro: This Greek Yogurt Parfait is a delightful combination of creamy Greek yogurt, crunchy nuts, and nutrient-rich seeds. It's a satisfying and wholesome breakfast that's easy to prepare.
Total Prep Time: 10 minutes

Ingredients:
- 1 cup Greek yogurt
- 1/4 cup granola
- 2 tablespoons mixed nuts (almonds, walnuts)
- 1 tablespoon chia seeds
- 1 tablespoon honey
- Fresh berries for topping

Instructions:
1. In a glass or bowl, layer Greek yogurt.
2. Add granola, mixed nuts, and chia seeds.
3. Drizzle honey over the layers.
4. Top with fresh berries.

Nutritional Information: (Per serving)
- Calories: 300
- Protein: 18g
- Carbohydrates: 25g
- Fiber: 5g
- Fat: 15g

Spinach and Feta Egg Muffins

Intro: These Spinach and Feta Egg Muffins are a convenient and protein-packed breakfast option. Packed with veggies and flavorful feta, they are perfect for a quick and healthy start to your day.

Total Prep Time: 25 minutes

Ingredients:
- 4 eggs
- 1 cup fresh spinach, chopped
- 1/2 cup feta cheese, crumbled
- 1/4 cup red bell pepper, diced
- Salt and pepper to taste
- Cooking spray

Instructions:
1. Preheat the oven to 350°F (175°C). Grease a muffin tin with cooking spray.
2. In a bowl, whisk eggs and season with salt and pepper.
3. Stir in chopped spinach, feta cheese, and diced red bell pepper.
4. Pour the mixture into muffin cups, filling each about two-thirds full.
5. Bake for 20 minutes or until the eggs are set.
6. Allow to cool slightly before serving.

Nutritional Information: (Per serving - 2 muffins)
- Calories: 220
- Protein: 15g
- Carbohydrates: 5g
- Fiber: 2g
- Fat: 16g

Overnight Chia Seed Pudding with Almond Milk

Intro: This Overnight Chia Seed Pudding is a make-ahead breakfast that's not only delicious but also packed with omega-3 fatty acids and fiber. Enjoy a nutritious and satisfying morning treat.

Total Prep Time: 5 minutes (plus overnight chilling)

Ingredients:
- 1/4 cup chia seeds
- 1 cup almond milk
- 1 tablespoon honey
- 1/2 teaspoon vanilla extract
- Fresh fruit for topping

Instructions:
1. In a jar or bowl, mix chia seeds, almond milk, honey, and vanilla extract.
2. Stir well and refrigerate overnight.
3. In the morning, give it a good stir and top with fresh fruit before serving.

Nutritional Information: (Per serving)
- Calories: 180
- Protein: 4g
- Carbohydrates: 20g
- Fiber: 10g
- Fat: 10g

Sweet Potato and Turkey Sausage Hash

Intro: This Sweet Potato and Turkey Sausage Hash is a hearty and flavorful breakfast option. Packed with protein and healthy carbohydrates, it's a satisfying dish to kickstart your day.

Total Prep Time: 30 minutes

Ingredients:
- 1 medium sweet potato, peeled and diced
- 1/2 pound turkey sausage, crumbled
- 1 bell pepper, diced
- 1 onion, chopped
- 2 cloves garlic, minced
- 1 teaspoon smoked paprika
- Salt and pepper to taste
- 2 tablespoons olive oil
- Fresh parsley for garnish (optional)

Instructions:
1. Heat olive oil in a skillet over medium heat.
2. Add diced sweet potatoes and cook until slightly tender.
3. Add turkey sausage, bell pepper, onion, and garlic. Cook until sausage is browned.
4. Season with smoked paprika, salt, and pepper.
5. Cook until sweet potatoes are fully cooked and slightly crispy.
6. Garnish with fresh parsley if desired.

Nutritional Information: (Per serving)
- Calories: 320
- Protein: 15g
- Carbohydrates: 25g
- Fiber: 5g
- Fat: 18g

Blueberry Almond Flour Pancakes

Intro: These Blueberry Almond Flour Pancakes are a gluten-free and nutritious twist on a classic breakfast favorite. With the goodness of almond flour and antioxidant-rich blueberries, they're a guilt-free delight.
Total Prep Time: 20 minutes

Ingredients:
- 1 cup almond flour
- 2 eggs
- 1/2 cup almond milk
- 1 tablespoon honey
- 1 teaspoon baking powder
- 1/2 teaspoon vanilla extract
- 1/2 cup blueberries

Instructions:
1. In a bowl, whisk together almond flour, eggs, almond milk, honey, baking powder, and vanilla extract.
2. Gently fold in blueberries.
3. Heat a griddle or non-stick pan over medium heat.
4. Pour batter onto the griddle to form pancakes.
5. Cook until bubbles form on the surface, then flip and cook the other side.
6. Serve with your favorite toppings.

Nutritional Information: (Per serving - 2 pancakes)
- Calories: 250
- Protein: 10g
- Carbohydrates: 20g
- Fiber: 5g
- Fat: 15g

Veggie Scramble with Tofu

Intro: This Veggie Scramble with Tofu is a plant-based breakfast option that's high in protein and bursting with flavor. It's a wholesome and satisfying way to start your day.

Total Prep Time: 15 minutes

Ingredients:
- 1/2 block firm tofu, crumbled
- 1/2 cup cherry tomatoes, halved
- 1/2 cup spinach, chopped
- 1/4 cup red onion, diced
- 1 clove garlic, minced
- 1 tablespoon nutritional yeast
- Salt and pepper to taste
- 1 tablespoon olive oil
- Fresh herbs for garnish (optional)

Instructions:
1. Heat olive oil in a pan over medium heat.
2. Add diced red onion and minced garlic. Sauté until softened.
3. Add crumbled tofu and cook until slightly golden.
4. Stir in cherry tomatoes and chopped spinach.
5. Season with nutritional yeast, salt, and pepper.
6. Cook until the vegetables are tender.
7. Garnish with fresh herbs if desired.

Nutritional Information: (Per serving)
- Calories: 230
- Protein: 15g
- Carbohydrates: 10g
- Fiber: 3g

- Fat: 15g

Salmon and Avocado Wrap

Intro: This Salmon and Avocado Wrap is a delicious and omega-3-rich option for a wholesome breakfast. Packed with protein and healthy fats, it's a filling and nutritious choice.

Total Prep Time: 15 minutes

Ingredients:
- 4 ounces smoked salmon
- 1 whole grain wrap
- 1/2 avocado, sliced
- 1/4 cup cucumber, thinly sliced
- 1 tablespoon cream cheese (optional)
- Fresh dill for garnish (optional)

Instructions:
1. Lay out the whole grain wrap.
2. Spread cream cheese if using.
3. Layer smoked salmon, sliced avocado, and cucumber.
4. Roll up the wrap tightly.
5. Slice in half and garnish with fresh dill if desired.

Nutritional Information: (Per serving)
- Calories: 300
- Protein: 20g
- Carbohydrates: 20g
- Fiber: 5g
- Fat: 15g

Oatmeal with Walnuts and Fresh Berries

Intro: This Oatmeal with Walnuts and Fresh Berries is a classic, heart-healthy breakfast option. Loaded with fiber, antioxidants, and omega-3 fatty acids, it's a comforting and nutritious way to start your day.

Total Prep Time: 15 minutes

Ingredients:
- 1/2 cup old-fashioned oats
- 1 cup milk (dairy or plant-based)
- 1/4 cup walnuts, chopped
- 1/2 cup mixed berries (strawberries, blueberries, raspberries)
- 1 tablespoon honey or maple syrup
- Dash of cinnamon (optional)

Instructions:
1. In a saucepan, bring the milk to a simmer.
2. Stir in the oats and cook until creamy.
3. Transfer to a bowl and top with chopped walnuts and mixed berries.
4. Drizzle with honey or maple syrup.
5. Sprinkle a dash of cinnamon if desired.

Nutritional Information: (Per serving)
- Calories: 280
- Protein: 10g
- Carbohydrates: 35g
- Fiber: 7g
- Fat: 12g

Cottage Cheese and Pineapple Bowl

Intro: This Cottage Cheese and Pineapple Bowl is a refreshing and protein-packed breakfast. The combination of creamy cottage cheese and sweet pineapple creates a tropical delight to kickstart your day.
Total Prep Time: 10 minutes

Ingredients:
- 1 cup low-fat cottage cheese
- 1 cup fresh pineapple chunks
- 1/4 cup unsweetened coconut flakes
- 1 tablespoon honey
- Mint leaves for garnish (optional)

Instructions:
1. In a bowl, spoon cottage cheese.
2. Top with fresh pineapple chunks.
3. Sprinkle unsweetened coconut flakes over the top.
4. Drizzle with honey.
5. Garnish with mint leaves if desired.

Nutritional Information: (Per serving)
- Calories: 220
- Protein: 15g
- Carbohydrates: 20g
- Fiber: 2g
- Fat: 10g

Whole Grain Toast with Smashed Avocado and Poached Egg

Intro: This Whole Grain Toast with Smashed Avocado and Poached Egg is a satisfying and nutritious breakfast option.

Packed with protein, healthy fats, and whole grains, it's a delicious way to start your day.
Total Prep Time: 15 minutes

Ingredients:
- 2 slices whole grain bread, toasted
- 1 ripe avocado, mashed
- 2 eggs, poached
- Salt and pepper to taste
- Red pepper flakes for garnish (optional)
- Chopped chives for garnish (optional)

Instructions:
1. Toast whole grain bread slices.
2. Spread mashed avocado evenly over each slice.
3. Top with a poached egg on each slice.
4. Season with salt and pepper.
5. Garnish with red pepper flakes and chopped chives if desired.

Nutritional Information: (Per serving)
- Calories: 320
- Protein: 15g
- Carbohydrates: 30g
- Fiber: 8g
- Fat: 18g

Berry Smoothie with Flaxseeds

Intro: This Berry Smoothie with Flaxseeds is a quick and delicious way to pack your morning with antioxidants, fiber, and essential fatty acids. It's a refreshing and nutrient-dense breakfast.
Total Prep Time: 10 minutes

Ingredients:
- 1 cup mixed berries (strawberries, blueberries, raspberries)
- 1 banana
- 1/2 cup Greek yogurt
- 1 tablespoon flaxseeds
- 1 cup almond milk
- Ice cubes (optional)
- Honey for sweetness (optional)

Instructions:
1. In a blender, combine mixed berries, banana, Greek yogurt, flaxseeds, and almond milk.
2. Blend until smooth and creamy.
3. Add ice cubes if desired and blend again.
4. Sweeten with honey if needed.
5. Pour into a glass and enjoy.

Nutritional Information: (Per serving)
- Calories: 250
- Protein: 10g
- Carbohydrates: 35g
- Fiber: 8g
- Fat: 8g

Zucchini and Mushroom Frittata

Intro: This Zucchini and Mushroom Frittata is a flavorful and veggie-packed breakfast option. Packed with protein and vitamins, it's a delicious way to incorporate more vegetables into your morning routine.

Total Prep Time: 25 minutes

Ingredients:

- 4 eggs
- 1 zucchini, sliced
- 1 cup mushrooms, sliced
- 1/2 onion, diced
- 1 clove garlic, minced
- 1/4 cup feta cheese, crumbled
- Salt and pepper to taste
- 1 tablespoon olive oil
- Fresh herbs for garnish (optional)

Instructions:

1. Preheat the oven to 350°F (175°C).
2. In an oven-safe skillet, heat olive oil over medium heat.
3. Add diced onion and minced garlic. Sauté until softened.
4. Add sliced zucchini and mushrooms. Cook until vegetables are tender.
5. In a bowl, whisk eggs and season with salt and pepper.
6. Pour the eggs over the vegetables in the skillet.
7. Sprinkle crumbled feta over the top.
8. Transfer the skillet to the preheated oven and bake for 15-20 minutes or until the eggs are set.
9. Garnish with fresh herbs if desired.

Nutritional Information: (Per serving)

- Calories: 280
- Protein: 15g
- Carbohydrates: 10g
- Fiber: 3g
- Fat: 20g

Almond Butter and Banana Sandwich

Intro: This Almond Butter and Banana Sandwich is a simple yet delicious breakfast option. Packed with protein, healthy fats, and natural sweetness, it's a satisfying way to start your day.

Total Prep Time: 10 minutes

Ingredients:
- 2 slices whole grain bread, toasted
- 2 tablespoons almond butter
- 1 banana, sliced
- Drizzle of honey (optional)
- Chia seeds for garnish (optional)

Instructions:
1. Toast whole grain bread slices.
2. Spread almond butter evenly over each slice.
3. Layer banana slices on one slice of bread.
4. Drizzle honey over the bananas if desired.
5. Sprinkle chia seeds on top.
6. Place the second slice of bread on top to create a sandwich.

Nutritional Information: (Per serving)
- Calories: 320
- Protein: 10g
- Carbohydrates: 45g
- Fiber: 8g
- Fat: 15g

Buckwheat Pancakes with Mixed Berries

Intro: These Buckwheat Pancakes with Mixed Berries offer a delicious twist on a classic breakfast favorite. The nutty flavor of buckwheat pairs perfectly with the sweetness of mixed berries for a wholesome and satisfying breakfast.

Total Prep Time: 25 minutes

Ingredients:
- 1 cup buckwheat flour
- 1 tablespoon sugar
- 1 teaspoon baking powder
- 1/2 teaspoon baking soda
- Pinch of salt
- 1 cup buttermilk
- 1 large egg
- 2 tablespoons melted butter
- Mixed berries for topping
- Maple syrup for serving

Instructions:
1. In a bowl, whisk together buckwheat flour, sugar, baking powder, baking soda, and salt.
2. In another bowl, whisk together buttermilk, egg, and melted butter.
3. Pour the wet ingredients into the dry ingredients and stir until just combined.
4. Heat a griddle or non-stick pan over medium heat.
5. Pour 1/4 cup of batter for each pancake onto the griddle.
6. Cook until bubbles form on the surface, then flip and cook the other side.
7. Top with mixed berries and serve with maple syrup.

Nutritional Information: (Per serving - 3 pancakes)
- Calories: 300
- Protein: 8g
- Carbohydrates: 45g
- Fiber: 6g
- Fat: 10g

Egg White and Spinach Breakfast Burrito

Intro: This Egg White and Spinach Breakfast Burrito is a protein-packed, low-fat option to kickstart your day. Filled with fluffy egg whites, vibrant spinach, and your favorite salsa, it's a flavorful and nutritious breakfast.

Total Prep Time: 15 minutes

Ingredients:
- 4 large egg whites
- 1 cup fresh spinach, chopped
- 1/4 cup diced tomatoes
- 2 tablespoons diced red onion
- 1/4 cup black beans, drained and rinsed
- 1 whole wheat tortilla
- Salsa for serving
- Avocado slices for garnish (optional)

Instructions:
1. In a non-stick pan, cook egg whites until fluffy.
2. Add chopped spinach, diced tomatoes, diced red onion, and black beans. Cook until vegetables are tender.
3. Warm the whole wheat tortilla.
4. Spoon the egg white and vegetable mixture onto the center of the tortilla.
5. Roll the tortilla into a burrito.

6. Serve with salsa and garnish with avocado slices if desired.

Nutritional Information: (Per serving)
- Calories: 220
- Protein: 20g
- Carbohydrates: 25g
- Fiber: 6g
- Fat: 5g

Greek Yogurt and Berry Smoothie Bowl

Intro: This Greek Yogurt and Berry Smoothie Bowl is a vibrant and nutrient-dense breakfast. Packed with protein from Greek yogurt and antioxidants from mixed berries, it's a delicious way to start your day.

Total Prep Time: 10 minutes

Ingredients:
- 1 cup Greek yogurt
- 1/2 cup mixed berries (strawberries, blueberries, raspberries)
- 1 banana, sliced
- 2 tablespoons granola
- 1 tablespoon chia seeds
- Drizzle of honey for sweetness (optional)

Instructions:
1. In a bowl, spread Greek yogurt as the base.
2. Arrange mixed berries and banana slices on top.
3. Sprinkle granola and chia seeds over the fruit.
4. Drizzle honey for sweetness if desired.
5. Serve immediately and enjoy with a spoon.

Nutritional Information: (Per serving)
- Calories: 300
- Protein: 20g
- Carbohydrates: 35g
- Fiber: 8g
- Fat: 10g

Walnut and Banana Oat Muffins

Intro: These Walnut and Banana Oat Muffins are a delightful combination of hearty oats, ripe bananas, and crunchy walnuts. They make for a wholesome and portable breakfast, perfect for those on the go.

Total Prep Time: 30 minutes

Ingredients:
- 1 cup old-fashioned oats
- 1 cup whole wheat flour
- 1 teaspoon baking powder
- 1/2 teaspoon baking soda
- Pinch of salt
- 2 ripe bananas, mashed
- 1/2 cup plain Greek yogurt
- 1/4 cup honey
- 1/4 cup melted coconut oil
- 1 large egg
- 1/2 cup chopped walnuts

Instructions:
1. Preheat the oven to 350°F (175°C). Line a muffin tin with paper liners.
2. In a bowl, combine oats, whole wheat flour, baking powder, baking soda, and salt.

3. In another bowl, mix mashed bananas, Greek yogurt, honey, melted coconut oil, and egg.
4. Pour the wet ingredients into the dry ingredients and stir until just combined.
5. Fold in chopped walnuts.
6. Spoon the batter into the muffin cups.
7. Bake for 20-25 minutes or until a toothpick comes out clean.
8. Allow to cool before serving.

Nutritional Information: (Per muffin)
- Calories: 180
- Protein: 5g
- Carbohydrates: 25g
- Fiber: 3g
- Fat: 8g

Veggie and Cheese Breakfast Quesadilla

Intro: This Veggie and Cheese Breakfast Quesadilla is a savory and satisfying option for a quick breakfast. Filled with colorful vegetables and gooey cheese, it's a delightful way to start your day.

Total Prep Time: 15 minutes

Ingredients:
- 1 whole wheat tortilla
- 1/2 cup shredded cheese (cheddar or Mexican blend)
- 1/4 cup bell peppers, diced
- 1/4 cup red onion, diced
- 1/4 cup tomatoes, diced
- 1/4 cup spinach, chopped
- 2 eggs, scrambled

- Salt and pepper to taste
- Salsa for serving
- Avocado slices for garnish (optional)

Instructions:
1. In a pan, cook scrambled eggs and season with salt and pepper.
2. Place the whole wheat tortilla in the pan over medium heat.
3. Sprinkle shredded cheese over half of the tortilla.
4. Add diced bell peppers, red onion, tomatoes, and chopped spinach on top of the cheese.
5. Spoon the scrambled eggs over the veggies.
6. Fold the tortilla in half, creating a semi-circle.
7. Cook until the cheese is melted and the tortilla is golden brown on both sides.
8. Serve with salsa and garnish with avocado slices if desired.

Nutritional Information: (Per serving)
- Calories: 350
- Protein: 20g
- Carbohydrates: 30g
- Fiber: 5g
- Fat: 18g

Cinnamon Raisin Oatmeal with Apples

Intro: This Cinnamon Raisin Oatmeal with Apples is a warm and comforting breakfast that combines the sweetness of apples with the warmth of cinnamon. It's a classic and nutritious way to start your day.

Total Prep Time: 15 minutes

Ingredients:
- 1/2 cup old-fashioned oats
- 1 cup milk (dairy or plant-based)
- 1/2 apple, diced
- 2 tablespoons raisins
- 1/2 teaspoon ground cinnamon
- 1 tablespoon honey or maple syrup
- Chopped nuts for garnish (optional)

Instructions:
1. In a saucepan, bring the milk to a simmer.
2. Stir in the oats, diced apples, raisins, and ground cinnamon.
3. Cook until the oats are tender and the mixture has thickened.
4. Sweeten with honey or maple syrup.
5. Top with chopped nuts if desired.
6. Serve warm and enjoy.

Nutritional Information: (Per serving)
- Calories: 280
- Protein: 8g
- Carbohydrates: 45g
- Fiber: 6g
- Fat: 8g

Avocado and Smoked Salmon Toast

Intro: This Avocado and Smoked Salmon Toast is a luxurious and nutrient-packed breakfast option. Creamy avocado, rich smoked salmon, and a touch of lemon create a delightful flavor combination that's perfect for a special morning treat.

Total Prep Time: 10 minutes

Ingredients:
- 2 slices whole grain bread, toasted
- 1/2 avocado, sliced
- 2 ounces smoked salmon
- Lemon wedge
- Fresh dill for garnish
- Salt and pepper to taste

Instructions:
1. Toast whole grain bread slices.
2. Spread sliced avocado evenly over each slice.
3. Lay smoked salmon over the avocado.
4. Squeeze a lemon wedge over the top.
5. Season with salt and pepper to taste.
6. Garnish with fresh dill.
7. Serve and enjoy your gourmet toast.

Nutritional Information: (Per serving)
- Calories: 300
- Protein: 15g
- Carbohydrates: 25g
- Fiber: 8g
- Fat: 15g

Tomato and Basil Quiche with Whole Wheat Crust

Intro: This Tomato and Basil Quiche with a Whole Wheat Crust is a delightful savory breakfast option. The combination of juicy tomatoes, fresh basil, and a whole wheat crust creates a flavorful and wholesome dish.

Total Prep Time: 40 minutes

Ingredients:
For the Crust:
- 1 cup whole wheat flour
- 1/2 cup cold unsalted butter, diced
- Pinch of salt
- 2-3 tablespoons ice water

For the Filling:
- 1 cup cherry tomatoes, halved
- 1/4 cup fresh basil, chopped
- 1 cup shredded mozzarella cheese
- 4 large eggs
- 1 cup milk (dairy or plant-based)
- Salt and pepper to taste

Instructions:
For the Crust:
1. In a food processor, combine whole wheat flour, cold diced butter, and a pinch of salt.
2. Pulse until the mixture resembles coarse crumbs.
3. Add ice water, one tablespoon at a time, until the dough comes together.
4. Shape the dough into a disk, wrap in plastic, and refrigerate for 30 minutes.
5. Roll out the chilled dough and press it into a pie dish.

For the Filling:
1. Preheat the oven to 375°F (190°C).
2. In a bowl, whisk together eggs, milk, salt, and pepper.
3. Sprinkle cherry tomatoes, chopped basil, and shredded mozzarella over the pie crust.
4. Pour the egg mixture over the fillings.

5. Bake for 25-30 minutes or until the quiche is set and golden brown.
6. Allow to cool slightly before slicing.

Nutritional Information: (Per serving)
- Calories: 320
- Protein: 15g
- Carbohydrates: 20g
- Fiber: 4g
- Fat: 20g

Green Tea Chia Seed Smoothie

Intro: This Green Tea Chia Seed Smoothie is a refreshing and antioxidant-rich beverage. Packed with the goodness of green tea and nutrient-dense chia seeds, it's a healthy and energizing way to start your day.
Total Prep Time: 10 minutes

Ingredients:
- 1 green tea bag
- 1 cup hot water
- 1 tablespoon chia seeds
- 1 banana
- 1 cup spinach leaves
- 1/2 cup pineapple chunks
- 1/2 cup almond milk
- Ice cubes (optional)
- Honey for sweetness (optional)

Instructions:
1. Steep the green tea bag in hot water and let it cool.

2. In a glass, mix chia seeds with the cooled green tea. Let it sit for 5-10 minutes until the chia seeds absorb the liquid and form a gel-like consistency.
3. In a blender, combine the chia seed mixture, banana, spinach, pineapple chunks, and almond milk.
4. Blend until smooth and creamy.
5. Add ice cubes if desired and blend again.
6. Sweeten with honey if needed.
7. Pour into a glass and enjoy your green tea chia seed smoothie.

Nutritional Information: (Per serving)
- Calories: 250
- Protein: 6g
- Carbohydrates: 40g
- Fiber: 8g
- Fat: 8g

Scrambled Tofu with Spinach and Tomatoes

Intro: This Scrambled Tofu with Spinach and Tomatoes is a protein-packed and plant-based breakfast option. Tofu, seasoned with spices and mixed with fresh vegetables, creates a flavorful and satisfying dish to kickstart your day.
Total Prep Time: 20 minutes

Ingredients:
- 1 block firm tofu, crumbled
- 1 cup fresh spinach, chopped
- 1 cup cherry tomatoes, halved
- 1/2 onion, diced
- 2 cloves garlic, minced

- 1 teaspoon turmeric powder
- 1/2 teaspoon cumin
- Salt and pepper to taste
- 1 tablespoon nutritional yeast (optional)
- 1 tablespoon olive oil
- Fresh herbs for garnish (optional)

Instructions:
1. Heat olive oil in a pan over medium heat.
2. Add diced onion and minced garlic. Sauté until softened.
3. Add crumbled tofu to the pan and cook until it starts to brown.
4. Sprinkle turmeric, cumin, salt, and pepper over the tofu. Mix well for even seasoning.
5. Stir in chopped spinach and halved cherry tomatoes.
6. Cook until the vegetables are wilted, and the tofu is well-cooked.
7. Optional: Add nutritional yeast for extra flavor and a cheesy touch.
8. Garnish with fresh herbs if desired.

Nutritional Information: (Per serving)
- Calories: 250
- Protein: 15g
- Carbohydrates: 10g
- Fiber: 5g
- Fat: 15g

Grilled Chicken Salad with Mixed Greens

Intro: This Grilled Chicken Salad with Mixed Greens is a vibrant and satisfying dish, perfect for a light and nutritious meal. Tender grilled chicken combines with a variety of fresh greens, creating a flavorful salad that's both delicious and wholesome.

Total Prep Time: 30 minutes

Ingredients:
- 2 boneless, skinless chicken breasts
- 6 cups mixed salad greens
- 1 cup cherry tomatoes, halved
- 1 cucumber, sliced
- 1/4 red onion, thinly sliced
- 1/2 cup crumbled feta cheese
- 1/4 cup balsamic vinaigrette dressing
- Salt and pepper to taste

Instructions:
1. Season chicken breasts with salt and pepper.
2. Grill the chicken until fully cooked, then slice it into strips.
3. In a large bowl, combine mixed greens, cherry tomatoes, cucumber, red onion, and grilled chicken.
4. Toss the salad with balsamic vinaigrette dressing.
5. Sprinkle crumbled feta cheese on top.
6. Serve immediately and enjoy this delightful grilled chicken salad.

Nutritional Information: (Per serving)
- Calories: 350
- Protein: 30g
- Carbohydrates: 15g
- Fiber: 5g
- Fat: 18g

Quinoa and Black Bean Bowl with Avocado

Intro: This Quinoa and Black Bean Bowl with Avocado is a wholesome and protein-packed meal that combines the goodness of quinoa, black beans, and creamy avocado. It's a delicious and nutritious option for those seeking a plant-based protein source.

Total Prep Time: 25 minutes

Ingredients:
- 1 cup quinoa, cooked
- 1 can black beans, drained and rinsed
- 1 cup corn kernels (fresh or frozen)
- 1/2 red bell pepper, diced
- 1/4 cup fresh cilantro, chopped
- 1 avocado, sliced
- Lime wedges for serving
- Salt and cumin to taste

Instructions:
1. In a bowl, combine cooked quinoa, black beans, corn, diced red bell pepper, and chopped cilantro.
2. Season with salt and cumin to taste, and mix well.
3. Serve in bowls, topping each with slices of avocado.
4. Garnish with lime wedges for a burst of citrus flavor.
5. Enjoy this nutrient-rich quinoa and black bean bowl.

Nutritional Information: (Per serving)
- Calories: 400
- Protein: 15g
- Carbohydrates: 55g
- Fiber: 12g

- Fat: 15g

Lentil Soup with Vegetables

Intro: This Lentil Soup with Vegetables is a hearty and nutritious option for a comforting meal. Packed with protein-rich lentils and a variety of vegetables, it's a flavorful soup that's both filling and wholesome.

Total Prep Time: 45 minutes

Ingredients:
- 1 cup dried green or brown lentils, rinsed
- 1 onion, diced
- 2 carrots, sliced
- 2 celery stalks, chopped
- 3 cloves garlic, minced
- 1 can diced tomatoes
- 6 cups vegetable broth
- 1 teaspoon cumin
- 1 teaspoon paprika
- Salt and pepper to taste
- Fresh parsley for garnish

Instructions:
1. In a large pot, sauté diced onion, sliced carrots, chopped celery, and minced garlic until softened.
2. Add dried lentils, diced tomatoes, vegetable broth, cumin, paprika, salt, and pepper.
3. Bring to a boil, then reduce heat and simmer until lentils are tender.
4. Adjust seasoning if necessary.
5. Garnish with fresh parsley before serving.
6. Enjoy this hearty lentil soup as a wholesome meal.

Nutritional Information: (Per serving)
- Calories: 280
- Protein: 18g
- Carbohydrates: 45g
- Fiber: 15g
- Fat: 2g

Turkey and Vegetable Wrap with Whole Grain Tortilla

Intro: This Turkey and Vegetable Wrap with Whole Grain Tortilla is a quick and delicious option for a balanced lunch. Packed with lean turkey, crisp vegetables, and wrapped in a whole grain tortilla, it's a satisfying and nutritious meal on the go.

Total Prep Time: 15 minutes

Ingredients:
- 4 whole grain tortillas
- 1 pound lean ground turkey
- 1 tablespoon olive oil
- 1 teaspoon taco seasoning
- 1 cup cherry tomatoes, halved
- 1 cup shredded lettuce
- 1/2 cup shredded cheddar cheese
- Greek yogurt or salsa for serving

Instructions:
1. In a skillet, heat olive oil and cook ground turkey until browned.
2. Season with taco seasoning and set aside.
3. Warm whole grain tortillas.
4. Assemble wraps by layering turkey, cherry tomatoes, shredded lettuce, and cheddar cheese.

5. Roll up the wraps and secure with toothpicks if needed.
6. Serve with Greek yogurt or salsa on the side.
7. Enjoy these flavorful turkey and vegetable wraps.

Nutritional Information: (Per serving - 1 wrap)
- Calories: 350
- Protein: 25g
- Carbohydrates: 30g
- Fiber: 5g
- Fat: 15g

Broccoli and Cheddar Stuffed Sweet Potato

Intro: This Broccoli and Cheddar Stuffed Sweet Potato is a delicious and nutrient-dense option for a wholesome meal. Roasted sweet potatoes are filled with a savory mixture of broccoli and melted cheddar cheese, creating a satisfying and flavorful dish.

Total Prep Time: 40 minutes

Ingredients:
- 4 medium-sized sweet potatoes
- 2 cups broccoli florets
- 1 cup shredded cheddar cheese
- 2 tablespoons olive oil
- Salt and pepper to taste
- Chopped chives for garnish (optional)

Instructions:
1. Preheat the oven to 400°F (200°C).
2. Scrub sweet potatoes, pierce them with a fork, and bake for 35-40 minutes or until tender.

3. In a pan, sauté broccoli florets with olive oil until slightly softened.
4. Cut a slit in each sweet potato and fluff the insides with a fork.
5. Stuff each sweet potato with sautéed broccoli and top with shredded cheddar.
6. Place the stuffed sweet potatoes back in the oven until the cheese melts.
7. Garnish with chopped chives if desired.
8. Enjoy this flavorful and nutritious stuffed sweet potato.

Nutritional Information: (Per serving)
- Calories: 300
- Protein: 10g
- Carbohydrates: 45g
- Fiber: 8g
- Fat: 12g

Greek Salad with Grilled Shrimp

Intro: This Greek Salad with Grilled Shrimp is a refreshing and protein-packed salad that combines the classic flavors of Greek cuisine. With crisp vegetables, feta cheese, olives, and succulent grilled shrimp, it's a delightful and satisfying meal.
Total Prep Time: 20 minutes

Ingredients:
- 1 pound large shrimp, peeled and deveined
- 2 tablespoons olive oil
- 1 teaspoon dried oregano
- 1 teaspoon garlic powder
- 6 cups mixed salad greens

- 1 cucumber, sliced
- 1 cup cherry tomatoes, halved
- 1/2 red onion, thinly sliced
- 1/2 cup feta cheese, crumbled
- Kalamata olives for garnish
- Greek dressing

Instructions:
1. In a bowl, marinate shrimp with olive oil, dried oregano, and garlic powder.
2. Grill shrimp until cooked through, about 2-3 minutes per side.
3. In a large salad bowl, combine mixed greens, cucumber, cherry tomatoes, and red onion.
4. Arrange grilled shrimp on top.
5. Sprinkle crumbled feta cheese and garnish with Kalamata olives.
6. Drizzle Greek dressing over the salad.
7. Toss gently and serve this delicious Greek salad with grilled shrimp.

Nutritional Information: (Per serving)
- Calories: 350
- Protein: 30g
- Carbohydrates: 15g
- Fiber: 5g
- Fat: 18g

Chickpea and Spinach Curry

Intro: This Chickpea and Spinach Curry is a flavorful and plant-based dish that's both satisfying and nutritious. With a rich blend of spices, chickpeas, and fresh spinach, it's a hearty curry that can be enjoyed with rice or naan.

Total Prep Time: 30 minutes

Ingredients:
- 2 cans chickpeas, drained and rinsed
- 1 onion, finely chopped
- 3 cloves garlic, minced
- 1 tablespoon ginger, grated
- 1 can diced tomatoes
- 1 can coconut milk
- 2 teaspoons curry powder
- 1 teaspoon turmeric
- 1 teaspoon cumin
- 1 teaspoon garam masala
- Salt and pepper to taste
- Fresh cilantro for garnish

Instructions:
1. In a pot, sauté chopped onion, minced garlic, and grated ginger until softened.
2. Add curry powder, turmeric, cumin, and garam masala. Stir until fragrant.
3. Pour in diced tomatoes and coconut milk. Bring to a simmer.
4. Add drained chickpeas and cook until heated through.
5. Fold in fresh spinach and cook until wilted.
6. Season with salt and pepper to taste.
7. Garnish with fresh cilantro before serving.
8. Enjoy this flavorful chickpea and spinach curry over rice or with naan.

Nutritional Information: (Per serving)
- Calories: 320
- Protein: 15g

- Carbohydrates: 40g
- Fiber: 12g
- Fat: 14g

Caprese Salad with Balsamic Glaze

Intro: This Caprese Salad with Balsamic Glaze is a classic and refreshing combination of ripe tomatoes, fresh mozzarella, and basil. Drizzled with a sweet balsamic glaze, it's a simple yet elegant dish that's perfect as a light lunch or appetizer.

Total Prep Time: 15 minutes

Ingredients:
- 4 large tomatoes, sliced
- 8 ounces fresh mozzarella, sliced
- Fresh basil leaves
- Balsamic glaze
- Extra virgin olive oil
- Salt and pepper to taste

Instructions:
1. Arrange sliced tomatoes and fresh mozzarella on a serving platter.
2. Tuck fresh basil leaves between the tomato and mozzarella slices.
3. Drizzle balsamic glaze and extra virgin olive oil over the salad.
4. Sprinkle with salt and pepper to taste.
5. Serve immediately and enjoy this simple and delicious Caprese Salad.

Nutritional Information: (Per serving)
- Calories: 250

- Protein: 15g
- Carbohydrates: 10g
- Fiber: 2g
- Fat: 18g

Grilled Vegetable and Hummus Wrap

Intro: This Grilled Vegetable and Hummus Wrap is a delightful and satisfying option for a plant-based lunch. Colorful grilled vegetables are wrapped in a whole grain tortilla, spread with creamy hummus, creating a flavorful and wholesome meal.
Total Prep Time: 30 minutes

Ingredients:
- 1 zucchini, sliced
- 1 red bell pepper, sliced
- 1 yellow bell pepper, sliced
- 1 red onion, sliced
- 2 tablespoons olive oil
- Salt and pepper to taste
- 4 whole grain tortillas
- 1 cup hummus
- Fresh spinach leaves

Instructions:
1. Preheat a grill or grill pan.
2. Toss sliced zucchini, red and yellow bell peppers, and red onion with olive oil, salt, and pepper.
3. Grill the vegetables until they are tender and slightly charred.
4. Warm whole grain tortillas.
5. Spread each tortilla with a generous layer of hummus.

6. Place a handful of fresh spinach leaves on each tortilla.
7. Top with grilled vegetables.
8. Roll up the wraps and secure with toothpicks if needed.
9. Enjoy these delicious grilled vegetable and hummus wraps.

Nutritional Information: (Per serving - 1 wrap)
- Calories: 320
- Protein: 10g
- Carbohydrates: 35g
- Fiber: 8g
- Fat: 18g

Salmon and Asparagus Foil Pack

Intro: This Salmon and Asparagus Foil Pack is a simple and nutritious dish that's easy to prepare. Fresh salmon fillets and tender asparagus are seasoned and baked in a foil pack, creating a flavorful and healthy meal.

Total Prep Time: 25 minutes

Ingredients:
- 4 salmon fillets
- 1 bunch asparagus, trimmed
- 2 tablespoons olive oil
- 1 lemon, sliced
- 2 cloves garlic, minced
- Fresh dill for garnish
- Salt and pepper to taste

Instructions:
1. Preheat the oven to 400°F (200°C).

2. Place each salmon fillet on a piece of foil large enough to fold into a packet.
3. Arrange trimmed asparagus around each salmon fillet.
4. Drizzle olive oil over the salmon and asparagus.
5. Season with minced garlic, salt, and pepper.
6. Place lemon slices on top of each salmon fillet.
7. Fold the foil into packets, sealing the edges.
8. Bake in the preheated oven for 15-20 minutes or until salmon is cooked through.
9. Garnish with fresh dill before serving.
10. Enjoy this flavorful and easy-to-make salmon and asparagus foil pack.

Nutritional Information: (Per serving)
- Calories: 350
- Protein: 30g
- Carbohydrates: 10g
- Fiber: 4g
- Fat: 20g

Quinoa and Roasted Vegetable Salad

Intro: This Quinoa and Roasted Vegetable Salad is a nutritious and satisfying dish that brings together the nuttiness of quinoa with the roasted goodness of a variety of vegetables. Packed with flavor and wholesome ingredients, this salad is an excellent option for a light and balanced meal.

Total Prep Time: 35 minutes

Ingredients:
- 1 cup quinoa, cooked
- 1 sweet potato, peeled and diced

- 1 zucchini, sliced
- 1 red bell pepper, chopped
- 1 yellow bell pepper, chopped
- 1 red onion, sliced
- 2 tablespoons olive oil
- 1 teaspoon dried thyme
- 1 teaspoon dried rosemary
- Salt and pepper to taste
- Balsamic vinaigrette dressing
- Fresh parsley for garnish

Instructions:

1. Preheat the oven to 425°F (220°C).
2. In a bowl, toss diced sweet potato, sliced zucchini, chopped red and yellow bell peppers, and sliced red onion with olive oil, dried thyme, dried rosemary, salt, and pepper.
3. Spread the vegetables on a baking sheet in a single layer.
4. Roast in the preheated oven for 20-25 minutes or until the vegetables are tender and slightly caramelized.
5. In a large bowl, combine cooked quinoa and the roasted vegetables.
6. Drizzle balsamic vinaigrette dressing over the salad and toss to coat.
7. Garnish with fresh parsley before serving.
8. Enjoy this flavorful and nutritious quinoa and roasted vegetable salad.

Nutritional Information: (Per serving)

- Calories: 300
- Protein: 8g
- Carbohydrates: 50g

- Fiber: 8g
- Fat: 10g

Turkey and Quinoa Stuffed Bell Peppers

Intro: These Turkey and Quinoa Stuffed Bell Peppers are a wholesome and protein-packed dish that combines lean ground turkey, quinoa, and a medley of vegetables. Baked to perfection, these stuffed peppers make for a satisfying and nutritious meal.

Total Prep Time: 50 minutes

Ingredients:
- 4 large bell peppers, halved and seeds removed
- 1 cup quinoa, cooked
- 1 pound lean ground turkey
- 1 onion, diced
- 2 cloves garlic, minced
- 1 can diced tomatoes, drained
- 1 cup black beans, drained and rinsed
- 1 teaspoon cumin
- 1 teaspoon chili powder
- Salt and pepper to taste
- 1 cup shredded cheddar cheese
- Fresh cilantro for garnish

Instructions:
1. Preheat the oven to 375°F (190°C).
2. Boil a pot of water and blanch the halved bell peppers for 3-5 minutes. Remove and set aside.
3. In a skillet, cook lean ground turkey until browned.
4. Add diced onion and minced garlic to the skillet and sauté until softened.

5. Stir in cooked quinoa, diced tomatoes, black beans, cumin, chili powder, salt, and pepper.
6. Fill each bell pepper half with the turkey and quinoa mixture.
7. Top with shredded cheddar cheese.
8. Bake in the preheated oven for 25-30 minutes or until the cheese is melted and bubbly.
9. Garnish with fresh cilantro before serving.
10. Enjoy these delicious and nutritious turkey and quinoa stuffed bell peppers.

Nutritional Information: (Per serving - 2 halves)
- Calories: 400
- Protein: 30g
- Carbohydrates: 35g
- Fiber: 8g
- Fat: 15g

Tofu and Vegetable Stir-Fry

Intro: This Tofu and Vegetable Stir-Fry is a quick and flavorful dish that combines tofu, colorful vegetables, and a savory stir-fry sauce. Packed with plant-based protein and vibrant flavors, it's a delightful and nutritious option for dinner.

Total Prep Time: 30 minutes

Ingredients:
- 1 block firm tofu, cubed
- 2 tablespoons soy sauce
- 1 tablespoon sesame oil
- 1 tablespoon cornstarch
- 2 tablespoons vegetable oil
- 1 bell pepper, sliced

- 1 carrot, julienned
- 1 cup broccoli florets
- 1 cup snap peas, trimmed
- 3 cloves garlic, minced
- 1 tablespoon ginger, grated
- Green onions for garnish
- Sesame seeds for garnish
- Cooked brown rice for serving

Instructions:
1. In a bowl, toss cubed tofu with soy sauce, sesame oil, and cornstarch until evenly coated.
2. Heat vegetable oil in a wok or large skillet over medium-high heat.
3. Add marinated tofu and cook until golden brown on all sides. Remove and set aside.
4. In the same pan, stir-fry sliced bell pepper, julienned carrot, broccoli florets, and snap peas until crisp-tender.
5. Add minced garlic and grated ginger to the vegetables and stir-fry for an additional minute.
6. Return the cooked tofu to the pan and toss everything together.
7. Serve over cooked brown rice.
8. Garnish with chopped green onions and sesame seeds.
9. Enjoy this flavorful tofu and vegetable stir-fry.

Nutritional Information: (Per serving)
- Calories: 350
- Protein: 15g
- Carbohydrates: 40g
- Fiber: 8g
- Fat: 18g

Spinach and Feta Turkey Burger

Intro: This Spinach and Feta Turkey Burger is a flavorful and lean option for a satisfying dinner. Ground turkey is mixed with spinach, feta cheese, and savory seasonings, creating a delicious and nutritious burger that's perfect for grilling.

Total Prep Time: 25 minutes

Ingredients:
- 1 pound lean ground turkey
- 1 cup fresh spinach, chopped
- 1/2 cup feta cheese, crumbled
- 1 clove garlic, minced
- 1 teaspoon dried oregano
- Salt and pepper to taste
- Whole grain burger buns
- Tzatziki sauce for serving
- Sliced tomatoes and lettuce for garnish

Instructions:
1. In a bowl, combine lean ground turkey, chopped fresh spinach, crumbled feta cheese, minced garlic, dried oregano, salt, and pepper.
2. Mix the ingredients until well combined.
3. Divide the mixture into burger-sized patties.
4. Grill the turkey burgers until fully cooked, about 4-5 minutes per side.
5. Toast whole grain burger buns on the grill.
6. Assemble the burgers with a spread of tzatziki sauce, a turkey patty, and garnish with sliced tomatoes and lettuce.
7. Serve these delicious spinach and feta turkey burgers.

Nutritional Information: (Per serving)
- Calories: 300
- Protein: 25g
- Carbohydrates: 30g
- Fiber: 5g
- Fat: 12g

Avocado and Black Bean Quesadilla

Intro: This Avocado and Black Bean Quesadilla is a quick and flavorful option for a meatless dinner. Creamy avocado, black beans, melted cheese, and a hint of spice are sandwiched between tortillas, creating a satisfying and delicious quesadilla.

Total Prep Time: 20 minutes

Ingredients:
- 4 whole wheat tortillas
- 1 can black beans, drained and rinsed
- 2 ripe avocados, sliced
- 1 cup shredded cheddar cheese
- 1 teaspoon cumin
- 1/2 teaspoon chili powder
- Salt and pepper to taste
- Olive oil for cooking
- Greek yogurt or salsa for serving

Instructions:
1. In a bowl, mash black beans with cumin, chili powder, salt, and pepper.
2. Spread the mashed black beans evenly over two of the whole wheat tortillas.
3. Top with sliced avocados and shredded cheddar cheese.

4. Place the remaining two tortillas on top to form quesadillas.
5. Heat olive oil in a skillet over medium heat.
6. Cook each quesadilla until the cheese is melted and the tortillas are golden brown, about 3 minutes per side.
7. Slice into wedges and serve with Greek yogurt or salsa on the side.
8. Enjoy these delicious avocado and black bean quesadillas.

Nutritional Information: (Per serving - 1 quesadilla)
- Calories: 350
- Protein: 12g
- Carbohydrates: 40g
- Fiber: 10g
- Fat: 15g

Minestrone Soup with Whole Wheat Pasta

Intro: This Minestrone Soup with Whole Wheat Pasta is a hearty and nutritious dish that brings together a medley of vegetables, beans, and whole wheat pasta. Bursting with flavors and packed with wholesome ingredients, it's a comforting soup perfect for any occasion.
Total Prep Time: 45 minutes

Ingredients:
- 1 cup whole wheat pasta, cooked
- 1 can kidney beans, drained and rinsed
- 1 cup diced carrots
- 1 cup diced celery
- 1 cup diced zucchini
- 1 onion, finely chopped

- 3 cloves garlic, minced
- 1 can diced tomatoes
- 6 cups vegetable broth
- 1 teaspoon dried oregano
- 1 teaspoon dried basil
- Salt and pepper to taste
- Fresh parsley for garnish
- Grated Parmesan cheese for serving (optional)

Instructions:
1. In a large pot, sauté onions and garlic until fragrant.
2. Add diced carrots, celery, and zucchini. Cook until slightly softened.
3. Pour in diced tomatoes and vegetable broth. Bring to a boil.
4. Stir in cooked whole wheat pasta, kidney beans, dried oregano, dried basil, salt, and pepper.
5. Simmer for 20-25 minutes until the vegetables are tender.
6. Adjust seasoning if necessary.
7. Garnish with fresh parsley and serve hot.
8. Optionally, sprinkle with grated Parmesan cheese.
9. Enjoy this wholesome Minestrone Soup!

Nutritional Information: (Per serving)
- Calories: 250
- Protein: 10g
- Carbohydrates: 45g
- Fiber: 8g
- Fat: 2g

Shrimp and Quinoa Spring Rolls

Intro: These Shrimp and Quinoa Spring Rolls are a refreshing and protein-packed twist on traditional spring rolls. Filled with succulent shrimp, quinoa, and crisp vegetables, they're served with a flavorful dipping sauce for a delightful appetizer or light meal.

Total Prep Time: 30 minutes

Ingredients:
- 12 spring roll rice wrappers
- 1 cup quinoa, cooked
- 1 pound shrimp, cooked and peeled
- 1 cucumber, julienned
- 1 carrot, julienned
- 1 avocado, sliced
- Fresh mint leaves
- Fresh cilantro leaves
- Rice vinegar for dipping sauce
- Soy sauce for dipping sauce
- Sesame oil for dipping sauce

Instructions:
1. Dip a rice wrapper into warm water until pliable.
2. Lay the wrapper flat and add a small portion of cooked quinoa.
3. Top with shrimp, cucumber, carrot, avocado, mint leaves, and cilantro.
4. Fold the sides of the wrapper and roll tightly.
5. Repeat with the remaining ingredients.
6. In a bowl, mix rice vinegar, soy sauce, and sesame oil for the dipping sauce.
7. Serve the spring rolls with the dipping sauce.

8. Enjoy these light and flavorful Shrimp and Quinoa Spring Rolls!

Nutritional Information: (Per serving - 2 spring rolls)
- Calories: 300
- Protein: 20g
- Carbohydrates: 40g
- Fiber: 6g
- Fat: 8g

Chicken Caesar Salad with Whole Grain Croutons

Intro: This Chicken Caesar Salad with Whole Grain Croutons is a wholesome take on the classic Caesar. Grilled chicken breast, crisp romaine lettuce, and whole grain croutons are tossed in a creamy Caesar dressing, creating a satisfying and nutritious salad.

Total Prep Time: 25 minutes

Ingredients:
- 2 boneless, skinless chicken breasts
- 1 head romaine lettuce, chopped
- 1 cup cherry tomatoes, halved
- 1/2 cup whole grain croutons
- 1/4 cup grated Parmesan cheese
- Caesar dressing (homemade or store-bought)
- Salt and pepper to taste
- Olive oil for grilling

Instructions:
1. Season chicken breasts with salt and pepper.
2. Grill the chicken until fully cooked, then slice into strips.

3. In a large bowl, combine chopped romaine lettuce, cherry tomatoes, whole grain croutons, and grilled chicken.
4. Toss the salad with Caesar dressing until well coated.
5. Sprinkle grated Parmesan cheese on top.
6. Serve immediately and enjoy this Chicken Caesar Salad with a wholesome twist.

Nutritional Information: (Per serving)
- Calories: 350
- Protein: 30g
- Carbohydrates: 20g
- Fiber: 5g
- Fat: 15g

Mediterranean Quinoa Salad

Intro: This Mediterranean Quinoa Salad is a vibrant and nutritious dish inspired by the flavors of the Mediterranean. Quinoa is mixed with colorful vegetables, olives, and feta cheese, then tossed in a lemony vinaigrette for a refreshing and wholesome salad.

Total Prep Time: 30 minutes

Ingredients:
- 1 cup quinoa, cooked
- 1 cup cherry tomatoes, halved
- 1 cucumber, diced
- 1 red bell pepper, diced
- 1/2 red onion, finely chopped
- 1/2 cup Kalamata olives, sliced
- 1/2 cup crumbled feta cheese
- Fresh parsley, chopped

- Lemon vinaigrette (olive oil, lemon juice, garlic, salt, and pepper)

Instructions:
1. In a large bowl, combine cooked quinoa, cherry tomatoes, cucumber, red bell pepper, red onion, Kalamata olives, and crumbled feta cheese.
2. In a separate small bowl, whisk together olive oil, lemon juice, minced garlic, salt, and pepper to create the lemon vinaigrette.
3. Pour the vinaigrette over the quinoa mixture and toss until well combined.
4. Garnish with fresh parsley.
5. Serve chilled and enjoy this Mediterranean Quinoa Salad.

Nutritional Information: (Per serving)
- Calories: 300
- Protein: 10g
- Carbohydrates: 35g
- Fiber: 6g
- Fat: 15g

Sweet Potato and Chickpea Buddha Bowl

Intro: This Sweet Potato and Chickpea Buddha Bowl is a nourishing and balanced meal that brings together roasted sweet potatoes, spiced chickpeas, and a variety of colorful vegetables. Drizzled with a tahini dressing, it's a flavorful and wholesome bowl that's easy to customize.

Total Prep Time: 40 minutes

Ingredients:
- 2 sweet potatoes, peeled and cubed

- 1 can chickpeas, drained and rinsed
- 1 tablespoon olive oil
- 1 teaspoon smoked paprika
- 1 teaspoon cumin
- 1 teaspoon garlic powder
- Salt and pepper to taste
- 4 cups mixed greens
- 1 avocado, sliced
- 1/2 cup shredded carrots
- 1/4 cup pumpkin seeds
- Tahini dressing (tahini, lemon juice, maple syrup, salt, and water)

Instructions:
1. Preheat the oven to 400°F (200°C).
2. Toss sweet potato cubes and chickpeas with olive oil, smoked paprika, cumin, garlic powder, salt, and pepper.
3. Roast in the preheated oven for 25-30 minutes or until golden brown and crispy.
4. In bowls, arrange mixed greens, roasted sweet potatoes, spiced chickpeas, avocado slices, shredded carrots, and pumpkin seeds.
5. In a small bowl, whisk together tahini, lemon juice, maple syrup, salt, and enough water to create a drizzle-worthy dressing.
6. Drizzle the tahini dressing over the Buddha bowls.
7. Serve and enjoy this delicious Sweet Potato and Chickpea Buddha Bowl.

Nutritional Information: (Per serving)
- Calories: 400
- Protein: 12g
- Carbohydrates: 45g

- Fiber: 10g
- Fat: 20g

Tomato Basil and Mozzarella Stuffed Chicken Breast

Intro: This Tomato Basil and Mozzarella Stuffed Chicken Breast is a flavorful and elegant dish that combines juicy chicken with the classic Caprese flavors. Baked to perfection, it's a delightful main course that's sure to impress.

Total Prep Time: 35 minutes

Ingredients:
- 4 boneless, skinless chicken breasts
- 1 cup cherry tomatoes, sliced
- 1/2 cup fresh basil leaves
- 1/2 cup fresh mozzarella, sliced
- 2 tablespoons balsamic glaze
- Salt and pepper to taste
- Olive oil for brushing

Instructions:
1. Preheat the oven to 375°F (190°C).
2. Butterfly each chicken breast to create a pocket for stuffing.
3. Season the inside of each chicken breast with salt and pepper.
4. Stuff each breast with sliced cherry tomatoes, fresh basil leaves, and mozzarella slices.
5. Close the pocket and secure with toothpicks if needed.
6. Place the stuffed chicken breasts in a baking dish.

7. Brush the tops with olive oil and sprinkle with additional salt and pepper.
8. Bake in the preheated oven for 25-30 minutes or until the chicken is cooked through.
9. Drizzle balsamic glaze over the stuffed chicken breasts before serving.
10. Enjoy this Tomato Basil and Mozzarella Stuffed Chicken Breast.

Nutritional Information: (Per serving)
- Calories: 350
- Protein: 40g
- Carbohydrates: 5g
- Fiber: 1g
- Fat: 18g

Spinach and Mushroom Whole Wheat Wrap

Intro: This Spinach and Mushroom Whole Wheat Wrap is a quick and nutritious lunch option filled with sautéed spinach and mushrooms, creamy feta cheese, and a flavorful tahini dressing. Wrapped in a whole wheat tortilla, it's a satisfying and wholesome meal.

Total Prep Time: 20 minutes

Ingredients:
- 1 cup baby spinach
- 1 cup mushrooms, sliced
- 1 clove garlic, minced
- 2 tablespoons feta cheese, crumbled
- 1 whole wheat tortilla
- Tahini dressing (tahini, lemon juice, garlic, salt, and water)

Instructions:
1. In a skillet, sauté sliced mushrooms and minced garlic until softened.
2. Add baby spinach to the skillet and cook until wilted.
3. Warm the whole wheat tortilla.
4. Place the sautéed spinach and mushrooms in the center of the tortilla.
5. Sprinkle crumbled feta cheese on top.
6. Drizzle with tahini dressing.
7. Fold the sides of the tortilla and roll it into a wrap.
8. Serve immediately and enjoy this Spinach and Mushroom Whole Wheat Wrap.

Nutritional Information: (Per serving)
- Calories: 250
- Protein: 8g
- Carbohydrates: 30g
- Fiber: 6g
- Fat: 12g

Brown Rice and Vegetable Sushi Bowl

Intro: This Brown Rice and Vegetable Sushi Bowl offers all the flavors of sushi in a convenient and customizable bowl. Brown rice is topped with a variety of fresh vegetables, avocado slices, and a drizzle of soy-ginger dressing for a delicious and wholesome meal.

Total Prep Time: 30 minutes

Ingredients:
- 2 cups brown rice, cooked
- 1 cucumber, julienned
- 1 carrot, julienned

- 1 avocado, sliced
- 1 cup edamame, shelled
- 1 nori sheet, crumbled
- Soy-ginger dressing (soy sauce, rice vinegar, ginger, garlic, and sesame oil)

Instructions:
1. Divide cooked brown rice among serving bowls.
2. Arrange julienned cucumber, carrot, avocado slices, shelled edamame, and crumbled nori sheet on top of the rice.
3. In a small bowl, whisk together soy sauce, rice vinegar, minced ginger, minced garlic, and sesame oil to create the dressing.
4. Drizzle the soy-ginger dressing over the sushi bowls.
5. Toss gently before enjoying this deconstructed Brown Rice and Vegetable Sushi Bowl.

Nutritional Information: (Per serving)
- Calories: 400
- Protein: 10g
- Carbohydrates: 60g
- Fiber: 8g
- Fat: 15g

Turkey and Vegetable Kebabs

Intro: These Turkey and Vegetable Kebabs are a flavorful and protein-packed option for a grilled meal. Lean ground turkey is mixed with vibrant vegetables, shaped onto skewers, and grilled to perfection. Served with a refreshing yogurt-based sauce, they make for a delicious and balanced dinner.

Total Prep Time: 40 minutes

Ingredients:
- 1 pound lean ground turkey
- 1 zucchini, sliced
- 1 red bell pepper, diced
- 1 red onion, sliced
- Cherry tomatoes
- Olive oil for brushing
- Salt and pepper to taste
- Wooden or metal skewers

Instructions:
1. Preheat the grill to medium-high heat.
2. In a bowl, mix lean ground turkey with salt and pepper.
3. Shape the turkey mixture onto skewers, alternating with zucchini slices, diced red bell pepper, red onion slices, and cherry tomatoes.
4. Brush the kebabs with olive oil.
5. Grill the kebabs for 12-15 minutes, turning occasionally, until the turkey is cooked through and the vegetables are charred.
6. Serve the Turkey and Vegetable Kebabs with your favorite sauce or dip.

Nutritional Information: (Per serving)
- Calories: 300
- Protein: 25g
- Carbohydrates: 15g
- Fiber: 4g
- Fat: 15g

Pesto Zoodles with Cherry Tomatoes

Intro: Pesto Zoodles with Cherry Tomatoes is a light and flavorful dish that replaces traditional pasta with spiralized zucchini. Tossed in a vibrant pesto sauce and garnished with sweet cherry tomatoes, it's a quick and healthy option for a satisfying meal.

Total Prep Time: 20 minutes

Ingredients:
- 4 medium-sized zucchini, spiralized
- 1 cup cherry tomatoes, halved
- 1/2 cup pine nuts, toasted
- 1/2 cup fresh basil leaves
- 1/2 cup grated Parmesan cheese
- 2 cloves garlic
- 1/2 cup extra-virgin olive oil
- Salt and pepper to taste
- Red pepper flakes for optional heat

Instructions:
1. Spiralize the zucchini into noodle-like strands.
2. In a food processor, combine fresh basil, toasted pine nuts, grated Parmesan cheese, garlic, salt, and pepper.
3. Pulse the ingredients while slowly adding the olive oil until a smooth pesto sauce forms.
4. In a large skillet, heat a small amount of olive oil over medium heat.
5. Add the zucchini noodles and sauté for 2-3 minutes until just tender.
6. Toss the zoodles with the prepared pesto sauce until well coated.
7. Add cherry tomatoes and toss gently to combine.

8. Garnish with additional Parmesan cheese and red pepper flakes if desired.
9. Serve immediately and savor the freshness of Pesto Zoodles with Cherry Tomatoes.

Nutritional Information: (Per serving)
- Calories: 350
- Protein: 8g
- Carbohydrates: 12g
- Fiber: 4g
- Fat: 30g

Baked Lemon Herb Salmon

Intro: This Baked Lemon Herb Salmon is a light and flavorful dish that showcases the natural goodness of salmon. The combination of zesty lemon, aromatic herbs, and tender salmon fillets creates a delightful and nutritious meal.

Total Prep Time: 25 minutes

Ingredients:
- 4 salmon fillets
- 2 tablespoons olive oil
- 2 tablespoons fresh lemon juice
- 1 teaspoon dried thyme
- 1 teaspoon dried rosemary
- Salt and pepper to taste
- Lemon slices for garnish
- Fresh parsley for garnish

Instructions:
1. Preheat the oven to 375°F (190°C).

2. Place salmon fillets on a baking sheet lined with parchment paper.
3. In a small bowl, mix olive oil, lemon juice, dried thyme, dried rosemary, salt, and pepper.
4. Brush the herb mixture over the salmon fillets.
5. Bake in the preheated oven for 15-20 minutes or until the salmon flakes easily with a fork.
6. Garnish with lemon slices and fresh parsley.
7. Serve this Baked Lemon Herb Salmon with your favorite sides.
8. Enjoy the light and citrusy flavors!

Nutritional Information: (Per serving)
- Calories: 300
- Protein: 25g
- Carbohydrates: 2g
- Fiber: 1g
- Fat: 20g

Eggplant and Chickpea Curry

Intro: This Eggplant and Chickpea Curry is a vibrant and hearty dish that brings together the rich flavors of eggplant, chickpeas, and aromatic spices. Simmered in a coconut milk-based curry sauce, it's a comforting and satisfying vegetarian curry.

Total Prep Time: 40 minutes

Ingredients:
- 1 large eggplant, diced
- 1 can chickpeas, drained and rinsed
- 1 onion, finely chopped
- 3 cloves garlic, minced
- 1 tablespoon curry powder

- 1 teaspoon ground cumin
- 1 teaspoon ground coriander
- 1 teaspoon turmeric
- 1 can coconut milk
- 1 can diced tomatoes
- Salt and pepper to taste
- Fresh cilantro for garnish
- Cooked rice for serving

Instructions:
1. In a large pot, sauté chopped onion and minced garlic until softened.
2. Add diced eggplant and cook until slightly browned.
3. Stir in curry powder, ground cumin, ground coriander, and turmeric.
4. Pour in coconut milk and diced tomatoes. Mix well.
5. Add chickpeas and simmer for 20-25 minutes until the eggplant is tender.
6. Season with salt and pepper to taste.
7. Garnish with fresh cilantro.
8. Serve over cooked rice and enjoy this Eggplant and Chickpea Curry.

Nutritional Information: (Per serving)
- Calories: 350
- Protein: 10g
- Carbohydrates: 40g
- Fiber: 12g
- Fat: 18g

Spaghetti Squash with Tomato and Basil Sauce

Intro: Spaghetti Squash with Tomato and Basil Sauce is a wholesome and low-carb alternative to traditional pasta. Roasted spaghetti squash strands are tossed in a flavorful tomato and basil sauce for a light and satisfying dish.
Total Prep Time: 50 minutes

Ingredients:
- 1 spaghetti squash, halved and seeded
- 2 tablespoons olive oil
- 1 onion, finely chopped
- 2 cloves garlic, minced
- 1 can crushed tomatoes
- 1/2 cup fresh basil, chopped
- 1 teaspoon dried oregano
- Salt and pepper to taste
- Grated Parmesan cheese for serving (optional)

Instructions:
1. Preheat the oven to 375°F (190°C).
2. Brush the cut sides of the spaghetti squash with olive oil and place them face down on a baking sheet.
3. Roast in the preheated oven for 40 minutes or until the squash is tender.
4. In a skillet, sauté chopped onion and minced garlic until fragrant.
5. Add crushed tomatoes, chopped fresh basil, dried oregano, salt, and pepper. Simmer for 10 minutes.
6. Use a fork to scrape the spaghetti squash strands into a bowl.

7. Toss the squash strands with the tomato and basil sauce.
8. Optional: Serve with grated Parmesan cheese on top.
9. Enjoy this light and flavorful Spaghetti Squash with Tomato and Basil Sauce!

Nutritional Information: (Per serving)
- Calories: 200
- Protein: 4g
- Carbohydrates: 30g
- Fiber: 7g
- Fat: 8g

Grilled Chicken with Rosemary and Garlic

Intro: Grilled Chicken with Rosemary and Garlic is a simple yet flavorful dish that highlights the classic combination of rosemary and garlic. The chicken is marinated, then grilled to perfection, creating juicy and aromatic chicken breasts.

Total Prep Time: 30 minutes (plus marinating time)

Ingredients:
- 4 boneless, skinless chicken breasts
- 3 tablespoons olive oil
- 2 tablespoons fresh rosemary, chopped
- 4 cloves garlic, minced
- 1 tablespoon lemon juice
- Salt and pepper to taste
- Lemon wedges for serving

Instructions:
1. In a bowl, mix olive oil, chopped rosemary, minced garlic, lemon juice, salt, and pepper.
2. Place chicken breasts in a resealable plastic bag or shallow dish and pour the marinade over them.
3. Marinate in the refrigerator for at least 2 hours, or overnight for maximum flavor.
4. Preheat the grill to medium-high heat.
5. Grill the chicken breasts for 6-8 minutes per side, or until fully cooked.
6. Let the chicken rest for a few minutes before slicing.
7. Serve with lemon wedges for an extra burst of flavor.
8. Enjoy this Grilled Chicken with Rosemary and Garlic as a tasty and protein-packed main course.

Nutritional Information: (Per serving)
- Calories: 250
- Protein: 30g
- Carbohydrates: 1g
- Fiber: 0g
- Fat: 13g

Cauliflower Fried Rice with Tofu

Intro: Cauliflower Fried Rice with Tofu is a delicious and low-carb alternative to traditional fried rice. Cauliflower rice is stir-fried with tofu, vegetables, and savory seasonings for a flavorful and satisfying dish.
Total Prep Time: 30 minutes

Ingredients:
- 1 medium cauliflower, riced

- 1 block firm tofu, pressed and cubed
- 2 tablespoons sesame oil
- 1 onion, finely chopped
- 2 carrots, diced
- 1 cup frozen peas
- 3 cloves garlic, minced
- 2 tablespoons soy sauce
- 1 teaspoon ginger, grated
- Green onions for garnish

Instructions:
1. Rice the cauliflower by using a food processor or grater.
2. Press the tofu to remove excess water, then cut it into cubes.
3. In a large skillet or wok, heat sesame oil over medium heat.
4. Add chopped onion, diced carrots, and cubed tofu. Stir-fry until the tofu is golden brown.
5. Add minced garlic, riced cauliflower, and frozen peas. Cook until the cauliflower is tender.
6. Pour soy sauce over the mixture and add grated ginger. Stir well.
7. Garnish with chopped green onions.
8. Serve this Cauliflower Fried Rice with Tofu as a flavorful and nutritious alternative to traditional fried rice.

Nutritional Information: (Per serving)
- Calories: 220
- Protein: 15g
- Carbohydrates: 15g
- Fiber: 6g
- Fat: 12g

Stuffed Bell Peppers with Quinoa and Black Beans

Intro: Stuffed Bell Peppers with Quinoa and Black Beans are a wholesome and protein-packed dish that combines the goodness of colorful bell peppers, quinoa, and black beans. Baked to perfection, these stuffed peppers are a satisfying and nutritious meal.

Total Prep Time: 45 minutes

Ingredients:
- 4 bell peppers, halved and seeds removed
- 1 cup quinoa, cooked
- 1 can black beans, drained and rinsed
- 1 cup corn kernels
- 1 cup diced tomatoes
- 1 cup shredded cheddar cheese
- 1 teaspoon chili powder
- 1/2 teaspoon cumin
- Salt and pepper to taste
- Fresh cilantro for garnish

Instructions:
1. Preheat the oven to 375°F (190°C).
2. In a bowl, mix cooked quinoa, black beans, corn kernels, diced tomatoes, shredded cheddar cheese, chili powder, cumin, salt, and pepper.
3. Stuff each bell pepper half with the quinoa and black bean mixture.
4. Place the stuffed peppers in a baking dish.
5. Bake in the preheated oven for 25-30 minutes or until the peppers are tender.
6. Garnish with fresh cilantro.

7. Serve these Stuffed Bell Peppers with Quinoa and Black Beans for a flavorful and colorful meal.

Nutritional Information: (Per serving - 2 stuffed pepper halves)
- Calories: 300
- Protein: 15g
- Carbohydrates: 40g
- Fiber: 8g
- Fat: 10g

Garlic and Herb Roasted Turkey Breast

Intro: Garlic and Herb Roasted Turkey Breast is a succulent and aromatic dish that's perfect for a festive dinner or any time you crave a flavorful turkey. The combination of garlic, herbs, and a golden-brown crust makes this turkey breast a delightful centerpiece.

Total Prep Time: 2 hours (includes marinating time)

Ingredients:
- 1 bone-in, skin-on turkey breast (about 4 pounds)
- 4 cloves garlic, minced
- 2 tablespoons fresh rosemary, chopped
- 2 tablespoons fresh thyme, chopped
- 1 tablespoon fresh sage, chopped
- 1/4 cup olive oil
- Salt and pepper to taste
- 1 cup chicken broth

Instructions:
1. Preheat the oven to 325°F (163°C).
2. Rinse the turkey breast and pat it dry with paper towels.

3. In a bowl, mix minced garlic, chopped rosemary, thyme, sage, olive oil, salt, and pepper.
4. Rub the garlic and herb mixture over the turkey breast, including under the skin.
5. Allow the turkey to marinate for at least 1 hour or overnight in the refrigerator.
6. Place the turkey breast in a roasting pan, and add chicken broth to the bottom.
7. Roast in the preheated oven for 1.5 to 2 hours, basting occasionally, until the internal temperature reaches 165°F (74°C).
8. Let the turkey breast rest for 15 minutes before carving.
9. Slice and serve this Garlic and Herb Roasted Turkey Breast as a flavorful and juicy main dish.

Nutritional Information: (Per serving)
- Calories: 350
- Protein: 40g
- Carbohydrates: 0g
- Fiber: 0g
- Fat: 20g

Zucchini Noodles with Pesto and Cherry Tomatoes

Intro: Zucchini Noodles with Pesto and Cherry Tomatoes is a light and refreshing dish that replaces traditional pasta with spiralized zucchini. Tossed in a vibrant pesto sauce and topped with sweet cherry tomatoes, it's a quick and healthy option for a satisfying meal.
Total Prep Time: 20 minutes

Ingredients:
- 4 medium-sized zucchini, spiralized
- 1 cup cherry tomatoes, halved
- 1/2 cup pine nuts, toasted
- 1/2 cup fresh basil leaves
- 1/2 cup grated Parmesan cheese
- 2 cloves garlic
- 1/2 cup extra-virgin olive oil
- Salt and pepper to taste
- Red pepper flakes for optional heat

Instructions:
1. Spiralize the zucchini into noodle-like strands.
2. In a food processor, combine fresh basil, toasted pine nuts, grated Parmesan cheese, garlic, salt, and pepper.
3. Pulse the ingredients while slowly adding the olive oil until a smooth pesto sauce forms.
4. In a large skillet, heat a small amount of olive oil over medium heat.
5. Add the zucchini noodles and sauté for 2-3 minutes until just tender.
6. Toss the zoodles with the prepared pesto sauce.
7. Add cherry tomatoes and toss gently to combine.
8. Garnish with additional Parmesan cheese and red pepper flakes if desired.
9. Serve immediately and savor the freshness of Zucchini Noodles with Pesto and Cherry Tomatoes.

Nutritional Information: (Per serving)
- Calories: 350
- Protein: 8g
- Carbohydrates: 12g
- Fiber: 4g

- Fat: 30g

Lentil and Vegetable Stew

Intro: Lentil and Vegetable Stew is a hearty and nutritious one-pot meal that brings together the earthy flavor of lentils with a variety of colorful vegetables. Simmered in a savory broth and aromatic spices, it's a comforting dish that's both filling and wholesome.

Total Prep Time: 50 minutes

Ingredients:
- 1 cup dried green or brown lentils, rinsed
- 1 onion, diced
- 2 carrots, sliced
- 2 celery stalks, chopped
- 3 cloves garlic, minced
- 1 can diced tomatoes
- 4 cups vegetable broth
- 1 teaspoon cumin
- 1 teaspoon smoked paprika
- 1/2 teaspoon turmeric
- Salt and pepper to taste
- Fresh parsley for garnish

Instructions:
1. In a large pot, sauté diced onion, sliced carrots, chopped celery, and minced garlic until softened.
2. Add dried lentils, diced tomatoes, vegetable broth, cumin, smoked paprika, turmeric, salt, and pepper. Stir well.
3. Bring the stew to a boil, then reduce the heat and simmer for 30-40 minutes or until the lentils are tender.

4. Adjust seasoning to taste.
5. Garnish with fresh parsley before serving.
6. Ladle this Lentil and Vegetable Stew into bowls for a comforting and protein-rich meal.

Nutritional Information: (Per serving)
- Calories: 300
- Protein: 18g
- Carbohydrates: 50g
- Fiber: 12g
- Fat: 2g

Baked Cod with Lemon and Dill

Intro: Baked Cod with Lemon and Dill is a light and flaky fish dish that's infused with the brightness of lemon and the aromatic touch of dill. This simple and healthy recipe lets the natural flavors of the cod shine through.
Total Prep Time: 20 minutes

Ingredients:
- 4 cod fillets
- 2 tablespoons olive oil
- Zest and juice of 1 lemon
- 2 tablespoons fresh dill, chopped
- 2 cloves garlic, minced
- Salt and pepper to taste
- Lemon wedges for serving

Instructions:
1. Preheat the oven to 400°F (200°C).
2. Place cod fillets in a baking dish.
3. In a bowl, mix olive oil, lemon zest, lemon juice, chopped dill, minced garlic, salt, and pepper.

4. Pour the lemon and dill mixture over the cod fillets, ensuring they are well-coated.
5. Bake in the preheated oven for 12-15 minutes or until the fish flakes easily with a fork.
6. Serve with lemon wedges for an extra burst of flavor.
7. Enjoy this Baked Cod with Lemon and Dill as a light and refreshing seafood option.

Nutritional Information: (Per serving)
- Calories: 250
- Protein: 30g
- Carbohydrates: 2g
- Fiber: 0g
- Fat: 13g

Sweet Potato and Black Bean Enchiladas

Intro: Sweet Potato and Black Bean Enchiladas are a delicious and satisfying vegetarian dish that combines the sweetness of roasted sweet potatoes with the savory goodness of black beans. Rolled in tortillas and baked with enchilada sauce, they're a flavorful and wholesome meal.
Total Prep Time: 1 hour

Ingredients:
- 2 large sweet potatoes, peeled and diced
- 1 can black beans, drained and rinsed
- 1 onion, finely chopped
- 2 cloves garlic, minced
- 1 teaspoon ground cumin
- 1 teaspoon chili powder
- 1/2 teaspoon smoked paprika
- Salt and pepper to taste

- 1 can enchilada sauce
- 8 whole wheat tortillas
- 1 cup shredded cheddar cheese
- Fresh cilantro for garnish
- Greek yogurt or sour cream for serving (optional)

Instructions:
1. Preheat the oven to 375°F (190°C).
2. Toss diced sweet potatoes with olive oil, salt, and pepper. Roast in the oven until tender.
3. In a skillet, sauté chopped onion and minced garlic until softened.
4. Add black beans, ground cumin, chili powder, smoked paprika, salt, and pepper. Cook until well combined.
5. Mix the roasted sweet potatoes with the black bean mixture.
6. Pour a small amount of enchilada sauce into the bottom of a baking dish.
7. Place a portion of the sweet potato and black bean filling in each whole wheat tortilla. Roll them and place them seam side down in the baking dish.
8. Pour the remaining enchilada sauce over the rolled tortillas.
9. Top with shredded cheddar cheese.
10. Bake in the preheated oven for 20-25 minutes or until the enchiladas are heated through and the cheese is melted and bubbly.
11. Garnish with fresh cilantro.
12. Serve these Sweet Potato and Black Bean Enchiladas with a dollop of Greek yogurt or sour cream if desired.

Nutritional Information: (Per serving - 2 enchiladas)
- Calories: 400

- Protein: 15g
- Carbohydrates: 60g
- Fiber: 12g
- Fat: 15g

Teriyaki Chicken Stir-Fry with Brown Rice

Intro: Teriyaki Chicken Stir-Fry with Brown Rice is a flavorful and wholesome dish that brings together tender pieces of chicken, vibrant vegetables, and a sweet and savory teriyaki sauce. Served over brown rice, it's a balanced and satisfying meal.

Total Prep Time: 30 minutes

Ingredients:
- 1 pound boneless, skinless chicken breasts, sliced
- 2 tablespoons soy sauce
- 2 tablespoons teriyaki sauce
- 1 tablespoon honey
- 1 tablespoon rice vinegar
- 1 tablespoon cornstarch
- 2 tablespoons vegetable oil
- 1 bell pepper, sliced
- 1 broccoli crown, cut into florets
- 1 carrot, julienned
- 2 cups cooked brown rice
- Sesame seeds and green onions for garnish

Instructions:
1. In a bowl, mix soy sauce, teriyaki sauce, honey, rice vinegar, and cornstarch to make the sauce.
2. In a wok or large skillet, heat vegetable oil over medium-high heat.

3. Add sliced chicken to the hot wok and stir-fry until browned and cooked through.
4. Remove the chicken from the wok and set aside.
5. In the same wok, add more oil if needed, and stir-fry bell pepper, broccoli, and julienned carrot until tender-crisp.
6. Return the cooked chicken to the wok and pour the teriyaki sauce over the chicken and vegetables. Stir to coat evenly.
7. Serve the Teriyaki Chicken Stir-Fry over cooked brown rice.
8. Garnish with sesame seeds and chopped green onions.
9. Enjoy this delicious and satisfying Teriyaki Chicken Stir-Fry with Brown Rice!

Nutritional Information: (Per serving)
- Calories: 400
- Protein: 25g
- Carbohydrates: 45g
- Fiber: 6g
- Fat: 15g

Quinoa-Stuffed Portobello Mushrooms

Intro: Quinoa-Stuffed Portobello Mushrooms are a flavorful and protein-packed vegetarian dish that showcases the robust taste of portobello mushrooms. Filled with a savory quinoa stuffing and baked to perfection, these mushrooms make for an elegant and nutritious meal.
Total Prep Time: 40 minutes

Ingredients:
- 4 large portobello mushrooms, stems removed

- 1 cup quinoa, cooked
- 1 onion, finely chopped
- 2 cloves garlic, minced
- 1 cup cherry tomatoes, halved
- 1/2 cup feta cheese, crumbled
- 1/4 cup fresh parsley, chopped
- 2 tablespoons balsamic glaze
- Salt and pepper to taste
- Olive oil for drizzling

Instructions:
1. Preheat the oven to 375°F (190°C).
2. Place portobello mushrooms on a baking sheet.
3. In a skillet, sauté chopped onion and minced garlic until softened.
4. Mix cooked quinoa with sautéed onion, garlic, cherry tomatoes, feta cheese, chopped fresh parsley, balsamic glaze, salt, and pepper.
5. Stuff each portobello mushroom cap with the quinoa mixture.
6. Drizzle olive oil over the stuffed mushrooms.
7. Bake in the preheated oven for 20-25 minutes or until the mushrooms are tender.
8. Serve these Quinoa-Stuffed Portobello Mushrooms as an elegant and nutritious dish.

Nutritional Information: (Per serving - 1 stuffed mushroom)
- Calories: 250
- Protein: 12g
- Carbohydrates: 35g
- Fiber: 6g
- Fat: 8g

Shrimp and Broccoli Quinoa Bowl

Intro: Shrimp and Broccoli Quinoa Bowl is a quick and flavorful dish that combines succulent shrimp, crisp broccoli, and fluffy quinoa. Tossed in a garlic and ginger-infused sauce, this bowl is a perfect balance of protein and veggies.

Total Prep Time: 30 minutes

Ingredients:
- 1 pound shrimp, peeled and deveined
- 1 cup quinoa, cooked
- 2 cups broccoli florets
- 3 cloves garlic, minced
- 1 tablespoon fresh ginger, grated
- 2 tablespoons soy sauce
- 1 tablespoon sesame oil
- 1 tablespoon honey
- Sesame seeds and green onions for garnish

Instructions:
1. In a large skillet or wok, heat sesame oil over medium-high heat.
2. Add shrimp and cook until pink and opaque. Remove shrimp from the skillet and set aside.
3. In the same skillet, add more sesame oil if needed, and stir-fry broccoli until tender-crisp.
4. Add minced garlic and grated ginger to the skillet. Cook for 1-2 minutes until fragrant.
5. Return the cooked shrimp to the skillet.
6. In a small bowl, mix soy sauce and honey. Pour the sauce over the shrimp and broccoli. Stir to coat evenly.

7. Serve the Shrimp and Broccoli Quinoa Bowl over cooked quinoa.
8. Garnish with sesame seeds and chopped green onions.
9. Enjoy this quick and tasty Shrimp and Broccoli Quinoa Bowl!

Nutritional Information: (Per serving)
- Calories: 350
- Protein: 25g
- Carbohydrates: 40g
- Fiber: 5g
- Fat: 10g

Ratatouille with Quinoa

Intro: Ratatouille with Quinoa is a delightful and colorful dish inspired by the classic French Provencal stew. This version adds protein-rich quinoa to the mix, creating a wholesome and satisfying meal that celebrates the flavors of seasonal vegetables.

Total Prep Time: 1 hour

Ingredients:
- 1 cup quinoa, cooked
- 1 eggplant, diced
- 2 zucchini, sliced
- 1 bell pepper, diced
- 1 onion, finely chopped
- 2 cloves garlic, minced
- 2 cups cherry tomatoes, halved
- 1 can crushed tomatoes
- 2 tablespoons tomato paste
- 1 teaspoon dried thyme

- 1 teaspoon dried rosemary
- Salt and pepper to taste
- Fresh basil for garnish

Instructions:
1. In a large pot, sauté diced eggplant, sliced zucchini, diced bell pepper, chopped onion, and minced garlic until softened.
2. Add cherry tomatoes, crushed tomatoes, tomato paste, dried thyme, dried rosemary, salt, and pepper. Stir well.
3. Simmer the ratatouille for 30-40 minutes, allowing the flavors to meld and the vegetables to become tender.
4. In the last 10 minutes of cooking, stir in the cooked quinoa.
5. Adjust seasoning to taste.
6. Serve this Ratatouille with Quinoa hot, garnished with fresh basil.
7. Enjoy the hearty and wholesome flavors of this vegetable-packed dish!

Nutritional Information: (Per serving)
- Calories: 300
- Protein: 10g
- Carbohydrates: 50g
- Fiber: 10g
- Fat: 5g

Lemon Garlic Herb Grilled Shrimp Skewers

Intro: These Lemon Garlic Herb Grilled Shrimp Skewers are a burst of fresh and zesty flavors. The succulent shrimp are marinated in a lemony garlic herb mixture, then grilled to perfection. This dish is perfect for a quick and flavorful seafood delight.

Total Prep Time: 20 minutes (plus marinating time)

Ingredients:
- 1 pound large shrimp, peeled and deveined
- 3 tablespoons olive oil
- 2 tablespoons fresh lemon juice
- 3 cloves garlic, minced
- 1 tablespoon fresh parsley, chopped
- 1 teaspoon dried oregano
- Salt and pepper to taste
- Lemon wedges for serving

Instructions:
1. In a bowl, mix olive oil, lemon juice, minced garlic, chopped parsley, dried oregano, salt, and pepper.
2. Add the shrimp to the marinade, ensuring they are well-coated. Marinate for at least 30 minutes.
3. Thread the marinated shrimp onto skewers.
4. Preheat the grill to medium-high heat.
5. Grill the shrimp skewers for 2-3 minutes per side or until they are opaque and grill marks appear.
6. Serve with lemon wedges for an extra citrus kick.
7. Enjoy these Lemon Garlic Herb Grilled Shrimp Skewers as a delightful appetizer or main course.

Nutritional Information: (Per serving)
- Calories: 200
- Protein: 25g
- Carbohydrates: 2g
- Fiber: 0g
- Fat: 10g

Mushroom and Spinach Stuffed Chicken Breast

Intro: Mushroom and Spinach Stuffed Chicken Breast is an elegant and savory dish that combines juicy chicken with a flavorful stuffing. The earthy mushrooms and tender spinach create a delicious filling, making this a perfect choice for a special dinner.

Total Prep Time: 40 minutes

Ingredients:
- 4 boneless, skinless chicken breasts
- 1 cup mushrooms, finely chopped
- 2 cups fresh spinach, chopped
- 1/2 cup feta cheese, crumbled
- 2 cloves garlic, minced
- 1 tablespoon olive oil
- 1 teaspoon dried thyme
- Salt and pepper to taste
- Toothpicks or kitchen twine for securing

Instructions:
1. Preheat the oven to 375°F (190°C).
2. In a skillet, sauté chopped mushrooms, minced garlic, and fresh spinach in olive oil until the spinach wilts.
3. Remove the skillet from heat and stir in crumbled feta, dried thyme, salt, and pepper.
4. Butterfly each chicken breast by slicing horizontally, creating a pocket without cutting all the way through.
5. Stuff each chicken breast with the mushroom and spinach mixture.

6. Secure the opening with toothpicks or kitchen twine.
7. Place the stuffed chicken breasts in a baking dish.
8. Bake in the preheated oven for 25-30 minutes or until the chicken is cooked through.
9. Remove toothpicks or twine before serving.
10. Enjoy this Mushroom and Spinach Stuffed Chicken Breast with your favorite side dishes.

Nutritional Information: (Per serving)
- Calories: 300
- Protein: 35g
- Carbohydrates: 4g
- Fiber: 2g
- Fat: 15g

Blackened Tilapia with Mango Salsa

Intro: Blackened Tilapia with Mango Salsa is a vibrant and flavorful dish that brings together the bold Cajun spices with the sweetness of fresh mango salsa. This combination creates a delicious contrast, making it a perfect light and healthy meal.

Total Prep Time: 30 minutes

Ingredients:
- 4 tilapia fillets
- 2 tablespoons Cajun seasoning
- 1 tablespoon olive oil
- 1 teaspoon paprika
- 1 teaspoon garlic powder
- 1 teaspoon onion powder
- Salt and pepper to taste

For Mango Salsa:
- 1 ripe mango, diced
- 1/2 red onion, finely chopped
- 1 jalapeño, seeded and minced
- 1/4 cup fresh cilantro, chopped
- Juice of 1 lime
- Salt to taste

Instructions:
1. In a bowl, mix Cajun seasoning, paprika, garlic powder, onion powder, salt, and pepper.
2. Rub the tilapia fillets with olive oil and coat them with the spice mixture.
3. Heat a skillet over medium-high heat.
4. Cook the tilapia fillets for 3-4 minutes per side or until blackened and cooked through.
5. In a separate bowl, combine diced mango, chopped red onion, minced jalapeño, chopped cilantro, lime juice, and salt to make the salsa.
6. Serve the Blackened Tilapia with Mango Salsa on top.
7. Enjoy the bold flavors of this delightful fish dish.

Nutritional Information: (Per serving)
- Calories: 250
- Protein: 30g
- Carbohydrates: 15g
- Fiber: 3g
- Fat: 8g

Veggie and Tofu Curry

Intro: Veggie and Tofu Curry is a comforting and nutritious dish that's rich in flavor and plant-based goodness. The combination of colorful vegetables, tofu, and aromatic spices creates a hearty curry that's perfect served over rice or with naan.

Total Prep Time: 45 minutes

Ingredients:
- 1 block firm tofu, pressed and cubed
- 2 tablespoons vegetable oil
- 1 onion, finely chopped
- 2 bell peppers, diced
- 1 zucchini, diced
- 1 cup cherry tomatoes, halved
- 1 cup broccoli florets
- 3 cloves garlic, minced
- 1 tablespoon ginger, grated
- 2 tablespoons curry powder
- 1 teaspoon ground cumin
- 1 teaspoon turmeric
- 1 can coconut milk
- Salt and pepper to taste
- Fresh cilantro for garnish

Instructions:
1. In a large skillet, heat vegetable oil over medium heat.
2. Add cubed tofu and cook until golden brown on all sides. Remove from the skillet and set aside.
3. In the same skillet, sauté chopped onion, bell peppers, zucchini, cherry tomatoes, and broccoli until softened.
4. Add minced garlic and grated ginger. Cook for 1-2 minutes until fragrant.
5. Stir in curry powder, ground cumin, and turmeric.

6. Pour in coconut milk and add the cooked tofu. Simmer for 15-20 minutes, allowing the flavors to meld.
7. Season with salt and pepper to taste.
8. Garnish with fresh cilantro before serving.
9. Serve this Veggie and Tofu Curry over rice or with naan for a satisfying plant-based meal.

Nutritional Information: (Per serving)
- Calories: 350
- Protein: 15g
- Carbohydrates: 20g
- Fiber: 6g
- Fat: 25g

Mediterranean Baked Eggplant

Intro: Mediterranean Baked Eggplant is a wholesome and flavorful dish inspired by the Mediterranean diet. Slices of eggplant are baked to perfection and topped with a delicious combination of tomatoes, olives, feta, and herbs. It's a delightful vegetarian option that captures the essence of Mediterranean cuisine.

Total Prep Time: 40 minutes

Ingredients:
- 2 large eggplants, sliced
- 2 tablespoons olive oil
- Salt and pepper to taste
- 1 cup cherry tomatoes, halved
- 1/2 cup Kalamata olives, sliced
- 1/2 cup feta cheese, crumbled
- 2 tablespoons fresh basil, chopped
- 1 tablespoon balsamic glaze (optional)

Instructions:
1. Preheat the oven to 375°F (190°C).
2. Place eggplant slices on a baking sheet.
3. Brush each slice with olive oil and season with salt and pepper.
4. Bake in the preheated oven for 20-25 minutes or until the eggplant is tender.
5. In a bowl, mix cherry tomatoes, Kalamata olives, feta cheese, and fresh basil.
6. Once the eggplant is done, top each slice with the tomato and olive mixture.
7. Drizzle with balsamic glaze if desired.
8. Serve this Mediterranean Baked Eggplant as a delightful and colorful side dish or appetizer.

Nutritional Information: (Per serving)
- Calories: 200
- Protein: 5g
- Carbohydrates: 15g
- Fiber: 7g
- Fat: 15g

Chicken and Vegetable Skewers with Yogurt Sauce

Intro: Chicken and Vegetable Skewers with Yogurt Sauce are a delicious and healthy option for a barbecue or a quick weeknight meal. The marinated chicken and colorful vegetables are threaded onto skewers and grilled to perfection, then served with a refreshing yogurt sauce.

Total Prep Time: 30 minutes (plus marinating time)

Ingredients:
- 1 pound boneless, skinless chicken breasts, cut into cubes
- 1 bell pepper, diced
- 1 red onion, diced
- 1 zucchini, sliced
- 1 cup cherry tomatoes
- 2 tablespoons olive oil
- 1 teaspoon smoked paprika
- 1 teaspoon cumin
- 1 teaspoon garlic powder
- Salt and pepper to taste

For Yogurt Sauce:
- 1 cup Greek yogurt
- 1 tablespoon fresh mint, chopped
- 1 tablespoon fresh cilantro, chopped
- 1 tablespoon lemon juice
- Salt and pepper to taste

Instructions:
1. In a bowl, mix olive oil, smoked paprika, cumin, garlic powder, salt, and pepper.
2. Marinate the chicken cubes in the spice mixture for at least 30 minutes.
3. Thread marinated chicken, bell pepper, red onion, zucchini, and cherry tomatoes onto skewers.
4. Preheat the grill to medium-high heat.
5. Grill the skewers for 10-12 minutes, turning occasionally, until the chicken is cooked through and the vegetables are tender.
6. In a separate bowl, mix Greek yogurt, chopped mint, chopped cilantro, lemon juice, salt, and pepper to make the yogurt sauce.

7. Serve the Chicken and Vegetable Skewers with Yogurt Sauce on the side.
8. Enjoy this flavorful and wholesome grilled dish!

Nutritional Information: (Per serving)
- Calories: 300
- Protein: 25g
- Carbohydrates: 15g
- Fiber: 3g
- Fat: 15g

Roasted Brussels Sprouts and Chicken Thighs

Intro: Roasted Brussels Sprouts and Chicken Thighs is a simple and satisfying one-pan dish that brings together the crispy goodness of roasted Brussels sprouts with juicy and flavorful chicken thighs. This recipe is easy to prepare and perfect for a hassle-free dinner.
Total Prep Time: 45 minutes

Ingredients:
- 4 bone-in, skin-on chicken thighs
- 1 pound Brussels sprouts, trimmed and halved
- 2 tablespoons olive oil
- 3 cloves garlic, minced
- 1 teaspoon dried thyme
- 1 teaspoon paprika
- Salt and pepper to taste
- Lemon wedges for serving

Instructions:
1. Preheat the oven to 425°F (218°C).

2. In a bowl, mix olive oil, minced garlic, dried thyme, paprika, salt, and pepper.
3. Place chicken thighs and Brussels sprouts on a baking sheet.
4. Brush the chicken thighs with the spice mixture, ensuring they are well-coated.
5. Roast in the preheated oven for 35-40 minutes or until the chicken is cooked through and the Brussels sprouts are crispy.
6. Serve with lemon wedges on the side for added freshness.
7. Enjoy this Roasted Brussels Sprouts and Chicken Thighs as a simple and delicious dinner option.

Nutritional Information: (Per serving)
- Calories: 400
- Protein: 30g
- Carbohydrates: 15g
- Fiber: 6g
- Fat: 25g

Butternut Squash and Kale Risotto

Intro: Butternut Squash and Kale Risotto is a comforting and hearty dish that combines the creamy goodness of risotto with the sweetness of butternut squash and the earthy flavor of kale. This vegetarian risotto is a perfect choice for a cozy and flavorful meal.

Total Prep Time: 50 minutes

Ingredients:
- 1 cup Arborio rice
- 1/2 cup dry white wine
- 4 cups vegetable broth

- 2 tablespoons olive oil
- 1 small onion, finely chopped
- 2 cloves garlic, minced
- 2 cups butternut squash, diced
- 2 cups kale, chopped
- 1/2 cup Parmesan cheese, grated
- Salt and pepper to taste

Instructions:

1. In a saucepan, heat vegetable broth over low heat. Keep it warm throughout the cooking process.
2. In a separate large pan, heat olive oil over medium heat.
3. Add chopped onion and garlic, sautéing until softened.
4. Stir in Arborio rice, ensuring each grain is coated with the oil and becomes slightly translucent.
5. Pour in the white wine, stirring continuously until absorbed by the rice.
6. Begin adding the warm vegetable broth one ladle at a time, stirring frequently. Allow the liquid to be absorbed before adding the next ladle. Continue this process until the rice is creamy and cooked to al dente, about 18-20 minutes.
7. In a separate skillet, sauté diced butternut squash until tender.
8. Add the cooked butternut squash and chopped kale to the risotto during the last 5 minutes of cooking. Stir well to incorporate.
9. Once the rice is cooked, stir in grated Parmesan cheese, and season with salt and pepper to taste.
10. Remove from heat and let it sit for a few minutes to allow the flavors to meld.

11. Serve this Butternut Squash and Kale Risotto warm, garnished with additional Parmesan if desired.

Nutritional Information: (Per serving)
- Calories: 400
- Protein: 10g
- Carbohydrates: 60g
- Fiber: 5g
- Fat: 12g

Baked Garlic Herb Chicken Thighs

Intro: Baked Garlic Herb Chicken Thighs are a simple yet flavorful dish that requires minimal effort. The combination of garlic and herbs creates a tasty coating for juicy chicken thighs, resulting in a delicious and easy-to-make main course.

Total Prep Time: 40 minutes

Ingredients:
- 4 bone-in, skin-on chicken thighs
- 4 cloves garlic, minced
- 2 tablespoons olive oil
- 1 tablespoon fresh rosemary, chopped
- 1 tablespoon fresh thyme, chopped
- 1 teaspoon paprika
- Salt and pepper to taste
- Lemon wedges for serving

Instructions:
1. Preheat the oven to 400°F (200°C).

2. In a small bowl, mix minced garlic, olive oil, chopped rosemary, chopped thyme, paprika, salt, and pepper.
3. Pat the chicken thighs dry with a paper towel.
4. Rub the garlic and herb mixture over the chicken thighs, ensuring they are well-coated.
5. Place the chicken thighs on a baking sheet, skin side up.
6. Bake in the preheated oven for 30-35 minutes or until the chicken is cooked through and the skin is crispy.
7. Serve with lemon wedges on the side for a zesty touch.
8. Enjoy these Baked Garlic Herb Chicken Thighs as a hassle-free and flavorful dinner option.

Nutritional Information: (Per serving)
- Calories: 350
- Protein: 25g
- Carbohydrates: 0g
- Fiber: 0g
- Fat: 28g

Quinoa and Black Bean Stuffed Acorn Squash

Intro: Quinoa and Black Bean Stuffed Acorn Squash is a nutritious and satisfying dish that showcases the natural sweetness of acorn squash. Filled with a hearty mixture of quinoa, black beans, and flavorful spices, this recipe is a delightful way to enjoy a wholesome and plant-based meal.
Total Prep Time: 1 hour

Ingredients:

- 2 acorn squash, halved and seeds removed
- 1 cup quinoa, cooked
- 1 can black beans, drained and rinsed
- 1 cup corn kernels (fresh or frozen)
- 1 bell pepper, diced
- 1 small red onion, finely chopped
- 2 cloves garlic, minced
- 1 teaspoon ground cumin
- 1 teaspoon chili powder
- 1/2 teaspoon smoked paprika
- Salt and pepper to taste
- 1/2 cup fresh cilantro, chopped
- Lime wedges for serving

Instructions:

1. Preheat the oven to 375°F (190°C).
2. Place acorn squash halves on a baking sheet, cut side down. Bake for 30-40 minutes or until the squash is tender.
3. In a skillet, sauté diced bell pepper, finely chopped red onion, and minced garlic until softened.
4. Add cooked quinoa, black beans, corn kernels, ground cumin, chili powder, smoked paprika, salt, and pepper to the skillet. Cook until well combined and heated through.
5. Remove the baked acorn squash from the oven. Fill each squash half with the quinoa and black bean mixture.
6. Garnish with chopped cilantro and serve with lime wedges on the side.
7. Enjoy this Quinoa and Black Bean Stuffed Acorn Squash as a wholesome and flavorful meal.

Nutritional Information: (Per serving)
- Calories: 350
- Protein: 12g
- Carbohydrates: 65g
- Fiber: 12g
- Fat: 5g

Printed in Great Britain
by Amazon

44402720R10059